Praise for

The Nurse Manager's Guide to an Intergenerational Workforce

66 The health care field has long predicted the day when members of the high-tech workforce become caregivers in a high-touch workplace. That day is now upon us. The generational differences that we see all around us in our daily lives are now alive in the nursing world, and Clipper does a remarkable job explaining the differences and bridging them in sound, well-thought-out ways. This book should be required reading for nurse managers; those who are most successful over the next 10 years will know how to effectively juggle generational differences. 99

–*Cam Marston*
President, Generational Insights

66 This highly practical resource will help nurse managers not only understand and relate to their multigenerational staff, but will also provide them with a unique source for communication that will help reduce conflict while increasing productivity. Ultimately, this information will help improve an organization's quality performance. I wish there had been a book like this when I first became a CNO! 99

–*Michael L. Evans, PhD, RN, NEA-BC, FACHE, FAAN*
Dean and Professor
Texas Tech University, Health Sciences Center, School of Nursing

" What Clipper has created in this book is a brilliantly practical work of art that transcends the generations and brings together both common wisdom and contemporary knowledge in a most enlightening way—one that is easily understood and, more importantly, easily translatable to the practice setting by leaders in any health profession. If you're looking for evidence-based leadership in the intergenerational space, this is THE book to have. From the pragmatic-ness of recruiting differences to the revelation that the generations are more the same than different—as it is value systems that shift, not ethics—this book has it all. A must-read for nurse leaders! "

–Cole Edmonson, DNP, RN, FACHE, NEA-BC
Vice President of Patient Care Services and Chief Nursing Officer
Texas Health Presbyterian Hospital Dallas
Robert Wood Johnson Foundation Executive Nurse Fellow

" Bonnie Clipper is the consummate professional nurse. Having successfully navigated the journey from staff nurse to chief nurse executive to Health System Excellence executive, she has experienced firsthand the challenges of our health care delivery system. She is one of few people equally qualified to provide guidance on meeting our health care challenges through fully engaging our intergenerational nursing workforce. This book is a must-read for not only nurse executives and nurse managers, but for all who are recruiting into and managing today's health care workforce. "

–Kenneth W. Dion, PhD, MSN, MBA, RN
Vice President, Healthstream

" Clipper's book provides today's managers with a useful tool for navigating the challenges of leading a multigenerational workforce. The book is grounded in research yet full of ready-to-use tools that managers will find directly applicable to everyday situations. "

–Jane Englebright, PhD, RN
Chief Nursing Officer and Vice President, HCA

" Without a doubt, the issue of professional 'dynamics' is one of the most important we are facing as a discipline. It speaks to how we work with and learn from each other; and as new graduates will tell you, the play-out of intraprofessional relationships in the workplace is one of THE most influential factors in the early transition experience to practice. I'm a baby boomer (primarily in age), and the last decade of working closely with Xers and millennials has brought to light how embedded generational understandings related to our work ethic, social conduct, and communication strongly impact how we engage in the workplace. Clipper's comprehensive resource for managers is both familiar and conversational, thereby easy to follow, while at once being strongly evidence-based and pragmatically structured. "

–Judy Boychuk Duchscher, PhD, RN
Author, From Surviving to Thriving: Navigating the First Year of
Professional Nursing Practice
Assistant Professor, University of Calgary, Alberta, Canada
Executive Director, Nursing the Future

" Uncovering the secret formula for nursing manager decision-making with an intergenerational workforce, Clipper helps leaders use generational culture's frame of reference to select, orient, communicate, assign, engage, and retain nurses. This guide will even help managers gauge the best way to motivate RNs in a staffing pinch! It's the bee's knees, groovy, cool, hot, and da bomb! "

–*Ruth Hansten, PhD, MBA, RN, FACHE*
Hansten Healthcare PLLC

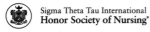

Sigma Theta Tau International
Honor Society of Nursing®

The Honor Society of Nursing, Sigma Theta Tau International (STTI), is a nonprofit organization whose mission is to support the learning, knowledge, and professional development of nurses committed to making a difference in health worldwide. Founded in 1922, STTI has 130,000 members in 86 countries. Members include practicing nurses, instructors, researchers, policymakers, entrepreneurs, and others. STTI's 486 chapters are located at 626 institutions of higher education throughout Australia, Botswana, Brazil, Canada, Colombia, Ghana, Hong Kong, Japan, Kenya, Malawi, Mexico, the Netherlands, Pakistan, Portugal, Singapore, South Africa, South Korea, Swaziland, Sweden, Taiwan, Tanzania, the United Kingdom, the United States, and Wales. More information about STTI can be found online at www.nursingsociety.org.

Sigma Theta Tau International
550 West North Street
Indianapolis, IN, USA 46202

To order additional books, buy in bulk, or order for corporate use, contact Nursing Knowledge International at 888.NKI.4YOU (888.654.4968/US and Canada) or +1.317.634.8171 (outside US and Canada).

To request a review copy for course adoption, e-mail solutions@nursingknowledge.org or call 888.NKI.4YOU (888.654.4968/US and Canada) or +1.317.634.8171 (outside US and Canada).

To request author information, or for speaker or other media requests, contact Rachael McLaughlin of the Honor Society of Nursing, Sigma Theta Tau International, at 888.634.7575 (US and Canada) or +1.317.634.8171 (outside US and Canada).

ISBN: 9781937554750
EPUB ISBN: 9781937554767
PDF ISBN: 9781937554774
MOBI ISBN: 9781937554781

Library of Congress Cataloging-in-Publication Data

Clipper, Bonnie.

The nurse manager's guide to an intergenerational workforce / Bonnie Clipper.
  p. ; cm.

Includes bibliographical references and index.

ISBN 978-1-937554-75-0 (print : alk. paper) -- ISBN 978-1-937554-76-7 (epub) -- ISBN 978-1-937554-77-4 (pdf) -- ISBN 978-1-937554-78-1 (mobi)

I. Sigma Theta Tau International. II. Title.

[DNLM: 1. Nursing--organization & administration. 2. Intergenerational Relations. 3. Interprofessional Relations. 4. Nurse's Role. 5. Nursing, Supervisory--organization & administration. WY 105]

610.73068--dc23

2012040296

First Printing, 2012

Publisher: Renee Wilmeth
Acquisitions Editor: Emily Hatch
Editorial Coordinator: Paula Jeffers
Copy Editor: Keith Cline
Cover Designer: Katy Bodenmiller
Interior Design & Page Layout: Katy Bodenmiller

Principal Book Editor: Carla Hall
Development Editor: Emily Hatch
Project Editor: Billy Fields
Proofreader: Heather Wilcox
Indexer: Jane Palmer
Illustrator: Aleata Halbig

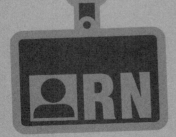

the NURSE MANAGER'S GUIDE to an INTER-GENERATIONAL WORKFORCE

Bonnie Clipper, DNP, MBA, MA, RN, CENP, FACHE

Sigma Theta Tau International
Honor Society of Nursing®

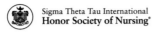

Sigma Theta Tau International
Honor Society of Nursing®

The Honor Society of Nursing, Sigma Theta Tau International (STTI), is a nonprofit organization whose mission is to support the learning, knowledge, and professional development of nurses committed to making a difference in health worldwide. Founded in 1922, STTI has 130,000 members in 86 countries. Members include practicing nurses, instructors, researchers, policymakers, entrepreneurs, and others. STTI's 486 chapters are located at 626 institutions of higher education throughout Australia, Botswana, Brazil, Canada, Colombia, Ghana, Hong Kong, Japan, Kenya, Malawi, Mexico, the Netherlands, Pakistan, Portugal, Singapore, South Africa, South Korea, Swaziland, Sweden, Taiwan, Tanzania, the United Kingdom, the United States, and Wales. More information about STTI can be found online at www.nursingsociety.org.

Sigma Theta Tau International
550 West North Street
Indianapolis, IN, USA 46202

To order additional books, buy in bulk, or order for corporate use, contact Nursing Knowledge International at 888.NKI.4YOU (888.654.4968/US and Canada) or +1.317.634.8171 (outside US and Canada).

To request a review copy for course adoption, e-mail solutions@nursingknowledge.org or call 888.NKI.4YOU (888.654.4968/US and Canada) or +1.317.634.8171 (outside US and Canada).

To request author information, or for speaker or other media requests, contact Rachael McLaughlin of the Honor Society of Nursing, Sigma Theta Tau International, at 888.634.7575 (US and Canada) or +1.317.634.8171 (outside US and Canada).

ISBN: 9781937554750
EPUB ISBN: 9781937554767
PDF ISBN: 9781937554774
MOBI ISBN: 9781937554781

Library of Congress Cataloging-in-Publication Data

Clipper, Bonnie.

  The nurse manager's guide to an intergenerational workforce / Bonnie Clipper.
    p. ; cm.

  Includes bibliographical references and index.

  ISBN 978-1-937554-75-0 (print : alk. paper) -- ISBN 978-1-937554-76-7 (epub) -- ISBN 978-1-937554-77-4 (pdf) -- ISBN 978-1-937554-78-1 (mobi)

  I. Sigma Theta Tau International. II. Title.

  [DNLM: 1. Nursing--organization & administration. 2. Intergenerational Relations. 3. Interprofessional Relations. 4. Nurse's Role. 5. Nursing, Supervisory--organization & administration. WY 105]

  610.73068--dc23

                2012040296

First Printing, 2012

Publisher: Renee Wilmeth
Acquisitions Editor: Emily Hatch
Editorial Coordinator: Paula Jeffers
Copy Editor: Keith Cline
Cover Designer: Katy Bodenmiller
Interior Design & Page Layout: Katy Bodenmiller

Principal Book Editor: Carla Hall
Development Editor: Emily Hatch
Project Editor: Billy Fields
Proofreader: Heather Wilcox
Indexer: Jane Palmer
Illustrator: Aleata Halbig

Dedication

This book is dedicated to my parents, Bob and Marilyn, and my kids, Sean and Ella. To my parents for their encouragement since age 6, providing the support for me to pursue every step of my nursing career. To my kids, who keep every day interesting and have kept it together while I have been busy working on this or that.

Acknowledgments

I would like to acknowledge and thank my family, friends, and colleagues for their support and confidence in me while I wrote this book.

A big thank you to my dad, Bob, and my kids, Sean and Ella, for putting up with me and finding creative ways to entertain themselves while I was writing. Who knew that you could do so many things with spare computer parts? And a big shout-out to my mom, Marilyn, who is watching this from above and wondering what is next for me. Stay tuned, Mom.

To:

Dr. Barbara Cherry and Dr. Alexia Green of Texas Tech University Health Sciences Center, School of Nursing, for their encouragement and support. Thank you for always making time for me.

Dr. Jo Stejskal of Winona State University, School of Nursing, for believing in me ever since I was a smart-%$# undergraduate nursing student. You rock!

Dr. Linda Yoder of the University of Texas at Austin, School of Nursing, for helping me think through everything so critically so I could see the big picture. Thank you for being such an excellent role model and mentor.

Bernie, thank you for being the only author friend I have and providing me with sound writing advice. I also have appreciated your being my cheerleader when I was tired of writing.

Kathy and Wendy, you guys are great friends and were able to support me through the fun parts and not-so-fun parts of getting myself into every new endeavor.

I also want to acknowledge everyone who has helped me along the way with this project.

About the Author

Bonnie Clipper, DNP, MBA, MA, RN, CENP, FACHE, is an experienced chief nursing officer, internal consultant, director, manager, and staff nurse. She is currently the associate vice president for Professional Nursing Practice and Development at St. David's HealthCare in Austin, Texas. Prior to this role, she was chief nursing officer for 12 years and has developed expertise in nursing leadership and direct patient care over the course of her career.

Clipper is the co-chair of the Central Texas Health Industry Steering Committee, which is an industry and academic collaboration that collectively addresses the workforce needs of the health care industry in the greater Austin metropolitan service area and surrounding communities. She serves on several nursing school and health care administration advisory boards. Additionally, she is actively involved with community organizations that are working toward building the nursing workforce pipeline. Because of her expertise, she has been called upon to provide expert testimony to the Texas State Senate regarding nursing issues.

In addition to her other responsibilities, Clipper is adjunct faculty for the University of Texas at Austin's School of Nursing, Texas Tech University Health Sciences Center's School of Nursing, and a guest lecturer at Winona State University's School of Nursing. She has been a grant reviewer for the state of Texas's higher education coordinating board and has extensive experience in educational, regulatory, and management processes as well as systems improvement and evaluation.

Clipper is a fellow in the American College of Health Care Executives and is certified in executive nursing practice. She received her Bachelor of Science in Nursing degree from Winona State University, her Master of Arts in Health and Human Services Administration from St. Mary's University, her Master of Business Administration from Lewis University, and her Doctor of Nursing Practice from Texas Tech University Health Sciences Center.

She is a full-blooded Gen Xer!

Table of Contents

Introduction

For many nurse managers, learning about generational differences is a fascinating topic that can be humorous. This is especially true as we see ourselves, friends, family, and even our staff in the generalizations we are so familiar with. Whether or not you find this topic too "fluffy" or lacking substance, you can't hide from the fact that many of the characteristics and attributes described in this book are visible in our current workforce. Understanding those traits and attitudes and why they exist will help you become a more effective nurse manager. Remember that these generalizations are based on patterns that have been observed over time comparing attitudes, values, behaviors, and life experiences. There are exceptions to these generalizations; not everyone has to fit a mold.

For the first time, four generations are working side by side, and three generations are leading the workplace. In any given organization, 20-year-olds through near-80-year-olds may be working in the same department. This fact is not unique to nursing, or even to health care; it is present in all industries. That span of 6 decades includes a very diverse group of people, with different attitudes, beliefs, values, goals, mores, and life experiences.

As a nurse manager, how do you meet everyone's needs and help them all become successful? How do you help your staff meet the needs of their patients, who are also likely to be of different generations? This book was written for the nurse manager as a tool book and guide to help improve your effectiveness and departmental performance.

Serious Business

The intergenerational workforce is a fun topic, but it is also important and relevant. One recent real-world example of the impact that multiple generations have in the workplace happened when a state nursing association sent a letter to all its members foreshadowing changes coming to the association (Texas Nurses Association, 2012). Although these changes are mostly due to the rapid rate of change in the current health care environment, the state nursing association referenced two leading reasons for changes to associations:

1. Full and busy lives

2. Generational differences

Figure I.1 is but one example of the relevance that this topic has taken on in our current environment.

Dear Member:

As your president, I am writing to communicate some potential changes for the future of our nurses association. Since we are all experiencing massive changes in health care and the profession of nursing, it is probably not surprising that change could potentially impact the American Nurses Association and the Texas Nurses Association.

Last summer, during the annual strategic planning process, the board of directors began a review of national trends in associations. As reference, we read two books suggested by the executive director: *Race for Relevance: 5 Radical Changes for Associations* by Harrison Coerver and Mary Byers, and *The End of Membership as We Know It: Building the Fortune-Flipping, Must-Have Association of the Next Century* by Sarah L. Sladek. Some key points they emphasize:

"Time—Americans are busier today than ever before. Their days are long; their calendars packed and schedules full. While all of this happens, associations continue with complicated governance and long meetings. We must change to capture our members."

"Generational Differences—a growing element of membership diversity falls along generational lines because for the first time in history, there are five living generations in America; four of these are in the workplace together. Each generation has its own values when it comes to volunteer service and the return on investment for their dues dollar."

Our analysis and our dialog assumed an urgent pace when the American Nurses Association announced initially to the leadership of its state affiliates that it would need to function within a very

different model if it was to remain the powerful national voice
of professional nursing. Even though the Board has examined,
considered and responded to the ANA information, it is now
imperative that in the coming weeks, the membership engage
in thoughtful participation to help determine what your future
professional nursing organization will be.

Our Nurses Association has been well managed over time and
is in fact one of the most financially independent state professional
nursing associations in the nation. For that, we owe our thanks to
our former Boards and our long-serving executive director and her
staff for this legacy and "gift," as it will enable the current Board and
members to have choices in determining what our future association
model might/should be.

FIGURE I.1
Texas Nurses Association newsletter.
(© 2012 Texas Nurses Association)

Although each generation has a "personality" that
is common to the generational cohort or group, it is
not safe to say that this personality can be generalized
or stereotyped. But there are common attributes and
characteristics that may be more pronounced in some
generations than in others.

Sure, times have changed, so what was taboo or
socially unacceptable in prior years or generations may be
acceptable now. But there are still some common themes
that run through a generation. As a nurse manager, you
should be able to identify these patterns and understand
how to customize your communication and leadership style
in a way that allows each generation to be successful and
fulfilled in the workplace. This will translate into higher
employee engagement, satisfaction, commitment, and ideally
a higher-functioning patient care team. The best metrics to
monitor this are employee turnover and engagement- as
well as exit-interview data (if your organization participates
in this). However, there are dangers in monitoring these

factors for this purpose. For example, the literature seems to indicate that in general there is less loyalty among millennials, which is often translated into higher turnover among this group. Ironically, our organization has found millennials to be the most satisfied group, based upon our employee engagement surveys. However, many organizations observe that their employee engagement/ satisfaction results indicate that although their millennials are more satisfied, as soon as they become dissatisfied, they just pick up and leave the organization, which is evidenced in turnover, especially among nurses.

Why Does It Matter?

Why is this topic important? Think of your staff. Imagine the training that the traditionalist or even baby boomer nurse received. How does it differ from the training that the Xer or millennial nurse received? How has technology changed patient care? How do your traditionalist nurses handle new technology? How do your millennial nurses handle conflict? How do your Xer nurses handle coaching? How do all your staff handle the amped-up expectations of customer service? Not only was the training different at various points in time, but each generation has different learning preferences, which means that the message was processed differently.

Although generational management is to some degree a "soft" science, there are clearly patterns among the attributes and characteristics that are common to each of these generations. Characteristics are not absolute for each generation, but rather collections of unique and distinctive traits. Although there is danger in stereotyping and over-generalizing, it is helpful to understand the generational differences so you can learn how to communicate in a way that the message you intended gets across to the audience as you planned. Be cautious and mindful of intragenerational differences of values, mores, and lifestyles. Remember, it is more likely that you will see many of the characteristics, but not necessarily all of them, in each person.

With four generations in the workplace at the same time, differences cannot be avoided. The goal is not to avoid the differences but rather to try to understand them and navigate through them for optimal outcomes. The generational "differences" that may occur though communication, style, or behavior are known as a "generation gap." These gaps are sometimes chasms and are evident through our collective differences in communication, dress, attitudes, work ethic, and even commitment (Felgen, 2001). The presence of generation gaps is frequently visible today due to the diverse nursing workforce. Your job as a nurse manager is to bridge the gaps.

Patient-Nurse Generation Gap

We know that there are age and thus generational differences among staff, but what happens when the nurse is a millennial and the patient is a traditionalist? It is more common than not for this to be the case. In fact, many misunderstandings have arisen from this simple scenario that repeats itself in every organization almost every day. For the millennial who enjoys multitasking, it seems as though he or she never quite has the time to sit calmly and at eye level with his or her patient for nurse-patient interactions. To the traditionalist patient this may seem rude and disrespectful, even though that is clearly not what was intended. However, the lack of being engaged and truly "present" in the conversation is not lost on our older patients and is often perceived as a lack of professionalism, a lack of knowledge, or a lack of enough time for the nurse never to talk to the patient.

Another patient-nurse gap is related to the fact that because many millennials have been raised more as their parents' "friend" than as their child, they have adopted a comfortable, casual style in their interactions between themselves and persons of "older" generations. This is uncomfortable for the traditionalists, as they have an expectation of formality and respect in their interactions. They prefer to be asked how they would like to be addressed—for example, "Hi Mr. Jones. I am Bonnie, your nurse for today. How would you like me to address you?" This provides the option for the patient to say, "Call me Bob," or "Call me Mr. Jones." Formality is something that Xers and millennials struggle with, while traditionalists and boomers expect it.

Another gap is technology. It cannot be overstated that both Xers and millennials are much more savvy and fearless with technology than boomers or traditionalists. The downside of this can be the patient's perception of this comfort level. Traditionalist patients may perceive that Xer and millennial nurses would rather deal with the machines and beeping alarms than address the patients, which is not necessarily true. However, traditionalist patients sense this and feel thwarted by it. This is yet one more reason why understanding the various generations is important, as is strong communication.

Physician-Nurse Generation Gap

The generation gap even creeps into interactions between nurses and physicians or other members of the health care team. Earlier we talked about millennials' being raised as their parents' friends and calling adults by their first names. Now translate that into the traditional health care environment. There are few limits among millennials, and often the informal use of first names is how millennials address physicians. As a young nurse, I would never have thought it acceptable to address a physician by his or her first name. That was just not done, so throughout my nursing career I have always spoken to or referred to physicians as "Dr. X" or "Dr. Y." However, our millennial nurses have no problem with first names. The casual nature of this interaction seems to be comfortable between late Xer and millennial physicians and nurses. But when an Xer or millennial nurse uses the first name of a boomer or traditionalist physician, you can see the hair on the back of his or her neck stand on end. Again there is no intended disrespect, so why is this regarded differently among the different generations?

These generational phenomena are not unique to nurses. As nurses share stories about notifying physicians regarding changes in patient conditions, it is not uncommon to hear stories about Xer or millennial physicians on the other end of the call. Often the nurse is greeted with "I am not on call," or "Talk to the on-call doctor." This is difficult for the boomer and traditionalist nurses to grasp, as this was not seen with the physicians of their generation, who were less adamant about not being on call. The "older" generation physicians accepted calls day and night to take care of their patients. Another scenario that highlights generational differences is when the traditionalist or late boomer physicians have a "favorite" nurse. Often these are nurses of or near their age with whom they have worked forever. On occasion, I have overheard some of these physicians say in their nicest indoor voices, "Where is Gail? I want her to take care of this patient. She has been here forever and knows how I like things." The unintended consequence of this is that it often offends millennial nurses, as they feel like they have already put in their time and should be seen in that light too. Or, worse yet, millennials may find it creepy or sexist. It is what it is. No harm. No foul. It is important to remember that everyone cannot be painted with the same generational brush.

A diverse workforce is part of our lives; that is the way it is. Do not fight it, resist it, or try to change it. Accept it, embrace it, understand it, and learn how to work with it. Today, nurse managers have to learn how to rise to the challenge of a workforce that has more ethnic, religious, gender, socioeconomic, age, and generational diversity than ever before. You just need to create harmony, a place where all your staff can flourish and patients will positively benefit. This is just one more challenge facing nursing managers, along with tight budgets, increased workload demands, increased satisfaction goals, and increased performance expectations.

Overview of the Chapters

This book consists of seven chapters, each one rich in information, tips, and tools. Due to the fun nature of this topic, this book is also interspersed with tips and anecdotes. The book has been organized to be as helpful to nurse managers as possible. The outline of the chapters is as follows:

Chapter 1: The Current Workforce—The goal of this chapter is to introduce the subject and provide examples of why this is a relevant and important topic. Although this is a "fluffy" topic, there are many recommendations that can improve the performance of the various generations. Nurse managers should be educated on strategies that work and pitfalls to avoid.

Chapter 2: Understanding the Generations—This chapter is intended to provide definitions, characteristics, and clarity regarding the different generations. The concept of a "cusper" is addressed along with differences in traditional social norms.

Chapter 3: Communication and Self-Expression—This chapter highlights the differences in written and verbal communication styles, use of social media, and how to best convey messages to each generation. This chapter also includes a section on body art as a means of self-expression and how it is perceived by coworkers and patients.

Chapter 4: Transition, Performance Management, and Succession Planning—This chapter tackles how to use preceptors in the orientation and transition process and how to establish and manage expectations. Training, learning preferences, coaching, action plans, and succession planning are also covered in this robust chapter.

Chapter 5: Recruitment and Retention Strategies—This chapter speaks to different tactics that are specific to each generation as it pertains to recruitment and hiring of new staff, including the application, interview process, and job-offer negotiations. This chapter also helps nurse managers establish a high-retention culture.

Chapter 6: How Does All This Impact the Patient?—This chapter considers everything previously explored about the four different generations and applies it to patient care, including patients and their relationships with their nurses and caregivers, health and wellness philosophies of each generation, and nurse-patient "pairing" or matching recommendations.

Chapter 7: Conclusions—This chapter provides a wrap-up of the topics discussed. You learn how to put all the pieces together and to integrate the information in order to be generationally fluent in communication.

I started my first chief nursing officer job at the age of 32 (remember, I am an Xer). I recall a situation when a family member came down to the executive offices and asked for the chief nursing officer (CNO). I was told about the family member and came out of my office to greet her and take her into a conference room where I could listen to her concerns. As I introduced myself to this very nice, traditionalist (65- to 70-year-old) woman, she was absolutely not satisfied with the fact that I was really the CNO. She asked me my age several times until I gave in and told her. She asked my administrative assistant to verify my name and title and even asked a house supervisor passing though to verify who I was. As a traditionalist, in her mind it was just not possible that I could hold the "rank" of CNO at what she felt was too young an age. That situation has since served as a reminder to me that it is important to fill in the blanks when introducing myself, such as saying, "Hi. I am Bonnie, the chief nursing officer at this facility. I have been a nurse for 25 years and have served in this capacity for 12 years." I have found that this helps in situations where age and/or generation may lead to different perceptions immediately upon introduction.

In writing this book, I wanted to make sure that it would be useful to nurse managers and serve as a tool to improve the way you communicate and accomplish your goals. Go ahead and highlight it, dog-ear it, and write all over it. The book is intended to help you understand generational differences and gain the awareness to help you become a better nurse manager. My intention is to help you learn how to harness generational strengths, which will help you become a more effective communicator and leader.

–Bonnie Clipper, DNP, MBA, MA, RN, CENP, FACHE

References

American Organization of Nurse Executives. (2012). Nurse Manager Leadership Partnership, Learning Domain Framework. Retrieved from http://www.aone.org/resources/leadership%20tools/NMLPframework.shtml

Coerver, H., & Byers, M. (2011). Race for relevance: 5 radical changes for associations. Washington, DC: ASAE: The Center for Association Leadership.

Felgen, J. (2001, September). *Dynamic dialogue: Application to generational diversity. Seminars for Nurse Managers, 9*(3), 164-168.

Karp, H., Fuller, C., & Sirias, D. (2002). Bridging the boomer-Xer gap: Creating authentic teams for high performance at work. Boston, MA: Davies-Black.

Lancaster, L., & Stillman, D. (2002). When generations collide. New York, NY: HarperCollins, Inc.

Sladek, S. (2011). The end of membership as we know it: Building the fortune-flipping, must-have association of the next century. Washington, DC: ASAE: The Center for Association Leadership.

Texas Nurses Association. (2012, April). Texas Nursing Magazine (member newsletter).

1

The Current Workforce

Each generation goes further than the generation preceding it because it stands on the shoulders of that generation. You will have opportunities beyond anything we've ever known.
–Ronald Reagan

Since first joining the nursing workforce, I have learned to recognize and to understand generational differences among staff, including why those differences exist. I just wish that I had understood them when I was a young nurse manager; back then, I didn't even know they existed. I was savvy enough to note differences among staff, but I usually attributed those differences merely to age. Many times I didn't understand why some staff "got it" while other staff didn't get it, or why some staff were more willing to help out the department and work extra shifts while other staff weren't willing to do so.

By taking the time to understand our current workforce, including their differences, we can more effectively communicate and optimize performance and thus better prepare not only nurse managers but also charge nurses, and even higher-level nurse leaders, to successfully accomplish their patient-care goals. After all, as a nurse manager you need to see the forest (the ultimate patient care) through the trees (staffing issues, including differences).

This chapter covers:

- Who makes up the current workforce
- Significance and implications of generational differences
- Understanding generational differences

Who Makes Up the Current Workforce?

Currently, four generations participate in the workforce:

- Traditionalists (the greatest generation/silent generation/veterans)
- Baby boomers (boomers)
- Generation X (Xers)
- Millennials (nexters, Gen Yers, echo boomers)

In addition to the four generations listed here, a not-yet-named generation is emerging.

Generational names are the handiwork of popular culture. Some draw their inspiration from a big event. Others relate to major social movements or demographic changes. A noteworthy turn in the calendar can also inspire a name.

The millennial generation falls into the third category. By our reckoning, the label covers everyone born from 1981 to 2000. It is the first generation to come of age in the new millennium.

The baby boomer label refers to the great spike in fertility that began in 1946, right after the end of World War II, and ended almost as abruptly in 1964, around the time that the birth control pill went on the market. It's a classic example of a demography-driven name.

The silent generation, sometimes known as the GI generation, covers anyone born before 1946. These are the children of the Great Depression and World War II. "Silent" overtook "GI" as the label relatively late in this generation's life cycle, when this group's conformist and civic instincts made for a dramatic contrast with the noisy ways of the antiestablishment boomers.

Generation X is a label that appears to have been coined by a British sociologist and popularized by author Douglas Coupland. It covers people born from 1965 to 1980, and it long ago overtook the first name affixed to this generation: the baby bust. In many generational profiles, Xers are depicted as savvy, entrepreneurial loners.

As these examples attest, generational names never stop being works in progress. The zeitgeist changes and labels that once seemed spot-on fall out of fashion. Millennials have also been described as Gen Yers or nexters. It's not clear if any of these three labels will stick—although a calendar change that comes along only once in 1,000 years feels like a pretty solid anchor.

© 2010 Pew Research Center

FIGURE 1.1

What's in a name?
(Pew Research Center, 2010)

Based on life experiences its members have shared, each generation has its own way of doing things and of viewing the world.

You have undoubtedly heard reports about the aging of the nursing population and how that affects the profession's numbers as older clinicians approach retirement. It also impacts the diversity currently represented within nursing. More than ever before, people from a wide range of age groups are working side by side within hospitals. Quite likely, this is the first time in history that four generations are participating in the workforce together, with three generations of leaders sharing the same workplace environment. The millennials are just beginning to assume leadership roles in larger numbers, too, and they will continue to fill leadership roles for many years to come. So, there are, or very soon will be, four generations of leaders in the workplace concurrently.

Generational differences are evident with regard to perceptions of authority, views of leadership, workplace relationships, thoughts on loyalty, and even what "turns them off" (Table 1.1).

The size of each generation has determined relative competition for opportunities in sports, education, and even jobs. In this past decade, for example, the college acceptance process has become extremely competitive, driving the growth of the cottage industry of consultants who assist with college applications or review courses to improve entrance exam scores. Competition was not as prevalent for Xers; there was no need for as much competition in a *smaller* generation.

Why Are We Talking About This?

As a nurse manager, you need to understand generational differences to optimize the performance of your team. Be aware, however, that those differences add another layer of complexity to the workplace. In addition to considering the diversity of religion, gender, culture, and race, a nurse manager needs to think about generational (not age) differences. Therefore, you have to become generationally fluent and a translator, able to communicate back and forth among the different generations.

TABLE 1.1
GENERATIONAL DIFFERENCES

	Size	Thoughts of Authority	Leadership Preference	Turnoffs	Loyalty To	Outlook	Relationships in the Workplace
Traditionalists	75 million	Respectful	Hierarchy	Vulgarity	Loyal to company/team	Practical	Don't have to like everyone
Boomers	80 million	Love/hate	Consensus	Politically incorrect	Loyal to my need to succeed	Optimistic	Get along and fit in
Xers	46 million	Unimpressed	Competent	Hype, lies	Loyal to individuals who help me with my career	Skeptical	Autonomous
Millennials	76 million	Polite	Pull team together	Promiscuity	Loyal to my need for meaningful work	Hopeful	Seek mentors. Large social network

(sourced from Alsop, 2008; Hicks & Hicks, 1999; Karp, 2001; Lancaster & Stillman, 2002; Meredith, Schewe, Hiam & Karlovich, 2002; Rich, 2008)

To effectively manage a nursing team and to lead a successful unit/department that provides the best patient care possible, you need to know which generations are represented on your staff and the characteristics, attributes, and needs of each of those generations.

Nursing presents various challenges, because the current workforce consists of approximately 5% traditionalists, 40% boomers, 40% Xers, and 15% millennials (Karp, 2001; Lancaster & Stillman, 2002). Buerhaus (2005) found that 24% of nurses were 22 to 34 years old, 48% of nurses were 35 to 49 years old, and 28% were 50 years old or older. No matter what data you look at, all indicate that we will lose seasoned nurses at a rapid pace starting in the not-too-distant future. The generational diversity we are experiencing adds complexity to the workplace— we're seeing traditionalists delaying retirement, boomers starting to retire, Xers realigning work/family priorities, and millennials who have a new set of demands for employers altogether (Rich, 2008). Nurse managers should see the multigenerational workforce as both an opportunity and a challenge. To succeed as a manager, you need to be more flexible and open-minded than ever.

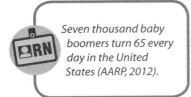

Seven thousand baby boomers turn 65 every day in the United States (AARP, 2012).

Having four different generations in the workforce means that generational differences will personally impact all of us in some form. The complexity of the current nursing workforce will also impact the organization as a whole. Possible organizational impacts include lack of employee commitment, increasing staff turnover, increasing patient complaints, dysfunctional teams, and working with functional disconnects (Rich, 2008). Although multigenerational differences might not seem significant, they play a crucial role in how expectations are set in the workplace. Each generation sees itself as unique.

> ### NOTE
>
> *To minimize tension on the unit, nurse managers need to learn how to interpret and ultimately deal with different styles of communication, frustration, anger, and discourse. Nurse managers also need to understand each group's worldview so as to comprehend its members perceptions and to focus on outcomes attainable by leveraging their strengths.*

The Changing Nursing Workforce

Not that long ago, health care authorities were planning for a sustained nursing shortage based on data that projected that by 2025, the national registered nurse (RN) workforce would fall short of demand by 260,000 nurses (Buerhaus, Staiger & Auerbach, 2009). The aging of the nursing workforce made it seem inevitable that increasingly large numbers of nurses would retire over the next several years. However, many factors, including the economic downturn of 2008, have mitigated this impact and have even had a positive effect on nursing workforce supply issues. A difficult economy has prompted many traditionalist and boomer nurses to postpone retirement, to return to nursing jobs, or to increase the number of nursing hours they work.

Offsetting the concern about impending retirements, an exciting trend has been building over the past decade. Nursing school output has increased, largely due to innovations in education and the increase in program sizes at schools across the country. This nursing student production trend has resulted in the growth of the overall

RN employment pool in recent years, and this trend consists, surprisingly, mostly of nurses 23 to 26 years old (millennials). The decline in the number of nurses in this age cohort witnessed in the 1980s and 1990s has since reversed, with a 62% increase in full-time equivalent RNs (Auerbach, Buerhaus & Staiger, 2011).

Collectively, these factors have seemingly mitigated the impact of nursing workforce supply issues. According to relevant data, the RN workforce is now projected to grow by 24% from 2009 to 2030. This is encouraging; it will allow the growth of the RN workforce to keep pace with the projected population growth over the same period. These recent findings suggest that as boomer nurses retire, they will, in fact, be replaced by even larger numbers of millennial nurses who are entering the profession, thus steadily increasing the size of the RN workforce (Auerbach et al., 2011). Great news, right? Absolutely! But are you prepared to manage the onslaught of millennial nurses entering the nursing workforce?

> **WHICH GENERATION IS THE MOST SOCIALLY CONSCIOUS?**
>
> Traditionalists 22%, boomers 34%, Xers 26 %, and millennials 19%. Harris Interactive survey of 3,868 adults ages 21–83 (Charles Schwab & Age Wave, 2008).

In 2008, the rate of aging of the nursing workforce slowed for the first time in 30 years (Buerhaus & Auerbach, 2011). In 1988, half the working RNs were younger than 38 years old (Buerhaus & Auerbach, 2011). By 2004, the median age rose to 46, but in 2008, the median age was still 46 (Buerhaus & Auerbach, 2011). That is good news, because there was fear that the median age would continue rising. From 2004 to 2008, the cohort of nurses under the age of 40 grew for the first time since the early 1980s (Buerhaus & Auerbach, 2011). In looking back at the 1980s, 54% of RNs were under the age of 40; by 1992, the percentage of RNs under the age of 40 had dropped to less than 45% (Buerhaus & Auerbach, 2011). This downward trend continued well into 2004, when the percentage of RNs under the age of 40 hit bottom at just under 27% (Buerhaus & Auerbach, 2011). By 2008, the percentage of RNs under the age of 40 was beginning to creep up to nearly 30% (Buerhaus & Auerbach). This was an increase of almost 18% over the 4 years since 2004. This positive trend related to the aging of the RN workforce resulted from an increase in the number of RNs younger than 30 years old (Buerhaus & Auerbach, 2011). The increase in the number of younger RNs is due to increasing enrollments in nursing programs, especially bachelor's degree programs (Buerhaus & Auerbach, 2011). This population is younger than those in previous initial nursing degree programs (Buerhaus & Auerbach). This trend in Bachelor of Science in Nursing (BSN) enrollment started years ago, and now these graduates are entering the workforce (Buerhaus & Auerbach). All of this is good news, because we will soon be experiencing large-scale reductions in hours or the retirement of our traditional and boomer nurses, not only bedside nurses but also nurse leaders.

Trends indicate that aging nurses become less and less likely to hold a nursing position (HRSA, 2010). This is demonstrated by the fact that 90% of nurses under the age of 50 are employed as nurses; 68% of those in the 50-54 age cohort—the second largest group—remain employed in nursing positions. However, by the time we get to nurses 65 years old and older, only 22% remain employed as nurses (HRSA, 2010). Not that long ago, health care authorities were planning for a sustained nursing shortage based on data that projected that by 2025, the national registered nurse (RN) workforce would fall short of demand by 260,000 nurses (Buerhaus, Staiger & Auerbach, 2009). The aging of the nursing workforce made it seem inevitable that increasingly large numbers of nurses would retire over the next several years. However, many factors, including the economic downturn of 2008, have mitigated this impact and have even had a positive effect on nursing workforce supply issues. A difficult economy has prompted many traditionalist and boomer nurses to postpone retirement, to return to nursing jobs, or to increase the number of nursing hours they work. Offsetting the concern about impending retirements, an exciting trend has been building over the past decade. Nursing school output has increased, largely due to innovations in education and the increase in program sizes at schools across the country. As discussed above, this nursing student production trend has resulted in the growth of the overall RN employment pool in recent years, and this trend consists, surprisingly, mostly of nurses 23 to 26 years old (millennials).

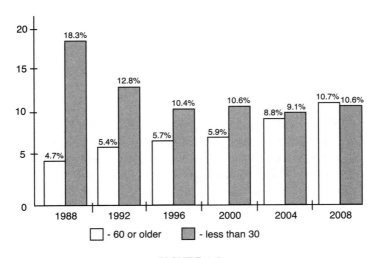

FIGURE 1.2
RNs by age, 1973-2009
(U.S. Bureau of Labor Statistics, n.d.; U.S. Census Bureau, n.d.)

Although training nurses in increasing numbers, especially younger nurses, to backfill those nurses who are retiring is important, it is also essential to improve retention. To minimize the impact on workforce supply, this equation has to be balanced on both sides, producing more nurses and retaining those we already have (see Figure 1.3). Although you'll not be able to eliminate turnover completely, you can and should reduce it. You can mitigate the impact of turnover by focused retention efforts (Wisotzkey, 2011).

> **NOTE**
>
> *To improve the work environment and to reduce turnover, nurse managers should focus appropriate time on job satisfaction, on engagement, and on managing generational expectations, social connectivity, and relationships on the unit. This is where nurse managers play a key role.*

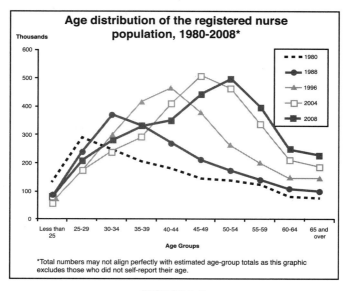

FIGURE 1.3
Percentage of hospital-employed RNs by age
(HRSA, 2010)

We have to get better at keeping new nurses. For newly graduated nurses, the transition to their new role is very important. Too often, however, the necessary time and resources required are not provided to smooth the transition and to make a lasting positive impression. Newly graduated nurses often describe themselves as overwhelmed as they transition from nursing student to nurse. Overcoming or minimizing these factors in the initial transition phase may increase retention of these newly graduated nurses. Generational differences also make a difference in managing both the needs and the expectations of newly graduated nurses. Younger nurses are more likely to leave in general, and therefore you need to consider this generational factor when planning aggressive retention goals or tactics (Wieck, Dols & Landrum, 2010; Wisotzkey, 2011).

NOTE

A word of advice for busy nurse managers: Focus on tactics that will meet the needs of the younger generations, such as flexible scheduling and opportunities that promote learning portable skills, if you are trying to retain them.

Over the years, many factors have influenced newly graduated nurse turnover. These factors include role transition, reality shock (Murphy, 2008), job satisfaction, pay, negative organizational environment, self-concept, horizontal violence (Bowles & Candela, 2005), relationships with coworkers, work environment, relationship with and support from manager, work rewards, organizational support and practices, physical and psychological responses to work, and patient relationships (Tourangeau, Cummings, Cranley, Ferron, & Harvey, 2010).

TABLE 1.2
GENERATIONAL PERCEPTIONS

	How Other Generations Perceive Them	How They Perceive Themselves
Traditionalists	Work too hard	Hard times just part of life
	Extremely loyal and committed	Able to sacrifice for "the cause"
	Will do what is right	Trustworthy and trusting
	Too willing to trust others	
Boomers	Need material goods	Hard working
	Ladder climbers	Play by the rules
	Need structure	Careful to trust authority
	Like process	Competitive
	Competitive	
Xers	Slackers	Self-absorbed
	Uncommitted	Independent (original latchkey kids)
	Short attention spans	Industrious
	Disloyal	Resourceful
	Arrogant	Value fun and balance
	Immature	Slow to commit to long-term relationships
	Poor social skills	Like feedback
		Risk takers
		Voracious learners
		Comfortable with diversity
		Just do it
Millennials	Have little respect for authority	Want to be led instead of managed
	Quit when they don't get their way	Want some say in decisions that affect them
	Entrepreneurial	Need personal attention
	Risk takers	Very tech savvy
	Lack of accountability	Want feedback
	Need constant praise and feedback	Want to be doing something meaningful
		Civic minded
		Major multitaskers

© *2010 Pew Research Center*

The goal of understanding the impact of generational differences is to create a work environment where generational harmony thrives. This doesn't mean that everyone has to walk around singing all shift; instead, it means managing a unit where staff learn to treat each other with respect and even cut their coworkers some slack on an ongoing basis. Harmony means that everyone can work together and have honest communication, use sensitivity when asking questions to better understand each generation, mentor, ask to be mentored, appreciate the differences, and respect each other's needs and feelings (Alsop, 2008). Think of how much more pleasant it is to work on a unit like this. Improving the level of understanding of generational differences among your staff sets the stage for improvements in turnover, customer service, and employee engagement. If you can make incremental improvements in those areas, imagine the quality of care that your patients can receive when all persons on your staff truly work like a satisfied and cohesive team.

> **TIP**
>
> *Young people today check the time on their cell phones. If you want to seem younger than you are, ditch the wristwatch (Satran, 2009).*

Summary

This chapter described the current workforce, including its characteristics and differences. Take the time to learn about generational differences so that you can improve the performance of your unit. It is also important to educate your unit leaders, such as charge nurses and shift supervisors, so that your staff will begin to understand generational differences. For example, you want them to know at least the basics: an introduction to the current workforce. Additionally, this chapter discussed the data on nurse production and who makes up the current workforce as well as the significance and implications of generational differences.

The time you spend learning about generational differences will help you build a high-performing team, establish respect, and create harmony among all your staff. This should pay off as increased employee engagement and improved patient care.

References

AARP. (2010). Approaching 65. Retrieved from http://www.aarp.org/personal-growth/transitions/info-12-2010/approaching-65.html

Alsop, R. (2008). *The trophy kids grow up*. San Francisco, CA. Jossey-Bass Publishing.

Auerbach, D. I., Buerhaus, P. I., & Staiger, D. O. (2011). Registered nurse supply grows faster than projected amid surge in new entrants ages 23-26. *Health Affairs*, *30*(12), 2286–2292.

Bowles, C., & Candela, L. (2005). First job experiences of recent RN graduates: Improving the work environment. *Nevada RNformation*, *14*(2), 16–19.

Buerhaus, P. I. (2005). Introduction: Six-part series on the state of the RN workforce in the United States. *Nursing Economics*, *23*(2), 58–61.

Buerhaus, P. I., Staiger, D. O., & Auerbach, D. A. (2009). The future of the nursing workforce in the United States: Data, trends and implications. Sudbury, MA. Jones and Bartlett Publishers.

Buerhaus, P. I., & Auerbach, D. I. (2011). The recession's effect on hospital registered nurse employment growth. *Nursing Economics*, *29*(4), 163–167.

Bureau of Labor Statistics (BLS). Retrieved from http://www.bls.gov/news.release/ecopro.t01.htm

Charles Schwab & Age Wave. (2008). Rethinking retirement: Four American generations share their views on life's third act. Retrieved from http://www.agewave.com/research/SchwabAgeWaveRethinkingRetirement071508.pdf

Hicks, R., & Hicks, K. (1999). *Boomers, X'ers and other strangers*. Wheaton, MD. Tyndale House Publishers.

HRSA. (2010). Retrieved from http://bhpr.hrsa.gov/healthworkforce/rnsurveys/rnsurveyfinal.pdf

Karp, H. F. (2001). *Bridging the boomer-X'er gap*. Palo Alto, CA. Davies-Black Publishing.

Keeter, S., & Taylor, P. (2009). The millennials. Pew Reserch Center Publications. Retrieved from http://pewresearch.org/pubs/1437/millennials-profile

Lancaster, L., & Stillman, D. (2002). *When generations collide*. New York, NY. Harper Business.

Meredith, G. E., Schewe, C. D., Hiam, A., & Karlovich, J. (2002). *Managing by defining moments*. New York, NY. Hungry Minds, Inc.

Murphy, B. E. (2008). Positive precepting: Preparation can reduce the stress. *MEDSURG Nursing, 17*(3), 183–188

Rich, P. (2008). HR management. Retrieved from http://www.hrmreport.com/article/Engaging-the-Multi-generational-Workforce

Satran, P. (2009). *How not to act old*. New York: HarperCollins Publishers.

Tourangeau, A. E., Cummings, G., Cranley, L. A., Ferron, E. M., & Harvey, S. (2010). Determinants of hospital nurse intention to remain employed: Broadening our understanding. *Journal of Advanced Nursing, 66*(1), 22–32.

Wieck, K. L., Dols, J., & Landrum, P. (2010). Retention priorities for the intergenerational nurse workforce. *Nursing Forum, 45*(1), 7–17.

Wisotzkey, S. (2011). Will they stay or will they go? Insight into nursing turnover. *Nursing Management, 42*(2), 15–17.

2

Understanding the Generations

*Our death is not an end if we can live on in our children
and the younger generation. For they are us, our bodies are
only wilted leaves on the tree of life.*

–Albert Einstein

A generation is defined generally by a period of time, a
series of events, and common icons, as well as by various
characteristics and attributes common to members of the
generation. These distinctions that help define a generation

often result in closer social interaction between those in the same generation as compared to intergenerational mingling. However, the workplace is one place where, on a regular basis, all the generations interact, with all their differences of opinion and insight.

For example, many Gen Xers and millennials think that baby boomers take their jobs and careers much too seriously; after all, where has it gotten them? Big houses, big cars, big debt. Boomers and traditionalists think, for the most part, that the Xers and millennials don't have a strong work ethic and give up too easily. (Boomers could be mentoring more, though. Perhaps where the Xers aren't receptive, the millennials are.) Millennials tend to have great relationships with their parents, who often raised this generation more as friends than as children. Although Xers like to work hard and play hard, they aren't willing to "pay the price" that their parents paid, as demonstrated by their reluctant (if any) loyalty and sense of commitment.

As a new generation begins to expand its role in the workplace, fostering an environment of understanding that values diversity will serve all of us well in the future. Because we seem to be healthier and working until later in life, generational differences in the work environment are here to stay.

NOTE

Understanding generational differences and learning how to communicate with and motivate each group is vital to a nurse manager's success.

This chapter covers:

- Each generation in the workforce today
- The generational differences in the workplace
- How each generation enters adulthood

What Defines a Generation?

Generally speaking, a generation is *not* an age. It is also *not* just a specific period of time. Instead, a generation is a cohort of individuals who have shared similar experiences (people, places, and events) and therefore often relate to the same things (Table 2.1). Similar values and common characteristics are obvious by-products of these shared experiences. Themes are apparent with regard to each generation, but it is important not to overgeneralize/ stereotype.

The word *generation* can be defined in several ways, including these three:

- An identifiable group that shares birth years, age, location, and significant life events at critical developmental stages

- A group of people who have shared filters, which are shared among those within the generation and allow them to interpret their experiences similarly

- A group is characterized by the historical, political, and social events that shape attitudes and values and are a revolution against the attitudes and values of the prior generation (Smola & Sutton, 2002; Wolburg & Pokrywczynski, 2001; Boychuk Duchscher & Cowin, 2004)

TABLE 2.1
SHARED PEOPLE, PLACES, AND EVENTS

	Traditionalists	Boomers	Xers	Millennials
People	Bob Hope	JFK	Michael Jordan	Tiger Woods
	Betty Crocker	Jackie O	Homer Simpson	Barack Obama
	Charles Lindbergh	MLK	Dilbert	George W. Bush
		Nixon	Bill Clinton	Dave Matthews
	John Wayne	The Beatles	Bill Gates	Eminem
	Hitler and Stalin	Rolling Stones	Madonna	Osama Bin Laden
	Elvis Presley	Charles Manson	Tom Cruise	OJ Simpson
	Frank Sinatra	Beat Generation	Michael Jackson	Ellen Degeneres
		Jimi Hendrix	Oprah	
Places	Pearl Harbor	Watergate Hotel	Somalia	New York City
	Normandy	Hanoi Hilton	Lockerbie	Afghanistan
	Iwo Jima	Chappaquiddick	Chernobyl	Iraq
		Woodstock		New Orleans
Events	Attack on Pearl Harbor	OPEC oil embargo	Berlin wall dismantling	Great Recession
	Invasion of Normandy	Women's rights movement	AIDS epidemic	Katrina
				Gulf Oil spill
	Battle of Iwo Jima	Civil rights movement	Assassination attempt on Pres. Reagan	Election of Pres. Barack Obama
	Korean War	Cuban missile crisis	Shooting of John Lennon	Oklahoma City bombing
	Great Depression	Bay of Pigs	1984 Summer Olympics	O.J. Simpson trial
	New Deal	Tet offensive		Death of Princess Diana
	GI Bill	Landing on the moon	Cold War	
Technology	Radio	Live TV	Cable TV	Mobile devices
	Mobile transportation	Computers	Home computers	Social networking
	Television		Gaming systems	
Defining Moment	WWI and WWII	Vietnam War	The shuttle *Challenger* explosion	9/11

Different authors use different years (time spans) to define each generation. I use the frequently cited Strauss and Howe (1991) parameters:

- Traditionalists (born 1925–1942)

- Boomers (1943–1960)

- Xers (1961–1981)

- Millennials (1982 to approximately 2000)

It looks like the latest generation began to be born around 2000 (or 2001), although this has not been "officially" determined yet.

WHAT IS A CUSPER?

You are a cusper if just one or two years separate you from another generation and you can relate to both generations. You are on the cusp of both generations. You can understand, relate to, appreciate, and likely display the behaviors, attitudes, and characteristics of both generations. You can knowledgably speak to and be an advocate for both generations. Cuspers make good peacekeepers. There are many of us out there.

Meet the Generations
Traditionalists (Silent Generation/ Greatest Generation/Matures)

Born between 1925 and 1942, this group is approximately 75 million strong. This group consists of two smaller groups: the GI generation (born 1901–1925) and the silent generation (1926–1945) (Strauss & Howe, 1991; Marston, 2010). These two groups are often characterized together in a larger group known as traditionalists. This group was shaped by the Great Depression, WWII, and the Korean War. They know hard work, hardship, and sacrifice. Such attributes as rules, law and order, patriotism, and faith are very important to this group. This group grew up in a "Norman Rockwell" world.

Traditionalists have impacted the workplace by setting the expectations. They are loyal, have a very strong work ethic, are willing to work toward a common goal and for the good of the group, and are currently the wealthiest generation (Marston, 2010). This generation is more comfortable with command-and-control leadership styles and looks to their leaders for direction and guidance. This group typically has only one career, believes in lifetime employment, and desires to have one or two employers over the course of their career. This group also tends to be uncomfortable with change in the workplace (Stanley, 2010).

As the traditionalists move out of the workforce, they are making room for the yet-to-be-named generation. This group is currently exhibiting a real dichotomy: Although its overall numbers are decreasing in the workforce (Figure 2.1), many who have left the workforce are (or will be) returning for financial reasons. The percentage of workers ages 75 and older in the workforce is projected to increase by 84% (over 2006 numbers) by 2016 (Figure 2.2). They are not returning to part-time jobs only; many are assuming full-time employment (Figure 2.3).

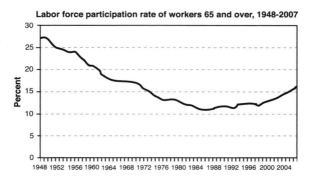

FIGURE 2.1
(2012. Bureau of Labor Statistics.)

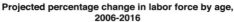

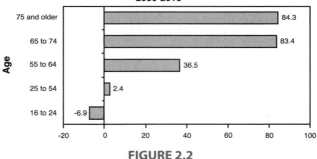

FIGURE 2.2
(2012. Bureau of Labor Statistics.)

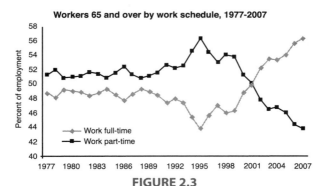

FIGURE 2.3
(2012. Bureau of Labor Statistics.)

Baby Boomers

Currently, the population of the baby boomers is about 80 million. This group was born between 1943 and 1960 (Strauss & Howe, 1991). Boomers were shaped by peace, love, and rock-n-roll. Well, officially, they were shaped by the equal rights movement and the Vietnam War.

As the boomers begin to retire, we will lose the largest portion of the current nursing workforce. As they leave, we lose not only a nurse but also untold years of experience, intuition, and expertise. This is hard to replace. When a new nurse fills a vacancy, that nurse takes years to develop the skills and expertise of a long-tenured nurse. As our boomer nurses age, we will experience a double-whammy: the loss of our most experienced workers at the same time that we experience an influx of new patients, the numbers of which will be larger than any we have seen before. Another factor we must consider is that as this group leaves the workforce, we will lose the majority of current nurse leaders and nurse executives. Who is going to fill all of those vacant positions? By default, Xers and millennials will fill those jobs.

THE SANDWICH GENERATION

Many boomers are currently experiencing what it's like to be the "sandwich generation," as many are taking care of their elderly parents while simultaneously welcoming their kids who have returned home from college back into the fold. This group is competitive and active, and it is likely to remain so well into retirement (think Sun City).

How have boomers impacted the workplace? Boomers like to work—in fact they "live to work," invented *workaholics*, and are especially satisfied when they perform well at work. They often spend energy on success-oriented goals, such as financial security, promotions, and a sense of accomplishment. Boomers are committed to their employers, are hard workers, and have a strong work ethic, which for them is measured in hours on the job. They are often viewed as *ladder climbers*, but they are patient and more than willing to put in the time it takes to move up or to be promoted. They invented the *corner office*. They currently compose the largest portion of the workforce, including executive and leadership positions.

Because they will live longer than their predecessors, boomers will need to work longer to adequately fund their retirements. To ensure the continuing efficacy of this group, modifications will need to be made en masse, such as shorter shifts, lifting teams, less-demanding nursing jobs, and so on. As a group, they generally have done a good job of accumulating wealth and want access to the *best* available, in every category. This generation pushes for answers and values the use of all available means for testing and treatment for themselves and their loved ones; this has, in part, contributed to higher health care costs.

Gen Xers

Born between 1961 and 1981 (Strauss & Howe, 1991), this is the smallest generational cohort (just 44 million). They are unique and leery of commitment, mostly because many are the children of divorce and have watched their parents get laid off. They were the original latchkey kids, many of whom wore a house key on a roller-skate shoelace around their neck so that they could let themselves and their siblings in after school (because both parents were working outside the home). I know that describes me as a kid.

This group has learned, out of necessity, to be fiercely independent, assertive, and industrious; they figure things out for themselves. Printed instructions were not made for this cohort; its members have no patience for them. This group hates process (which boomers just love). They want to "just do it" and get it done and strongly prefer outcomes over tenure (Marston, 2010).

Twenty-four-hour cable television was the new thing for them, replacing the television stations going off-air at midnight. (I wish I could count the times I awoke to TV "snow" and the sound of static as a kid when I was allowed to stay up and watch television late on Friday nights.) This group is also very well-traveled (loves travel) and values individualism. This group truly needs constant exposure to information (for example, CNN, Twitter, online news sources). This is the generational cohort that as consumers has demanded value from the marketplace. This group has introduced second-career nurses to the profession.

It can be tough being an Xer. Older Xers, just like many boomers, are truly experiencing the sandwich generation, which is tiring and exhausting for this group. Worrying about raising their children, who might even be of college age, as well as their parents, who are well into the traditionalist generation, is taxing for them. Whereas 6 in 10 Xers indicate that it is their responsibility to move their parents into their own homes to take care of them, only 4 in 10 traditionalists feel this way (Pew Research Center, 2010). Ironically, this might be welcome news for these Xers.

How has this group affected the workplace? It isn't as though this group doesn't have a strong work ethic. However, Xers are known to work to live, not live to work. As a whole, Xers tend to be loyal to themselves but not necessarily to the organization. In fact, they often see loyalty as a temporary condition, depending on what's in it for them. This group also strongly values work-life balance; this becomes evident when talking about working off-shifts, holidays, or taking calls. There is not much acceptance of

the *greater good* or of *the whole* at this point, but rather
a preference for the good of the individual. As employees,
they need to know exactly what is expected of them and
what the benefits are before they proceed so that they
can decide whether it's worth it for them to participate
(Marshburn & Scott, 2009). Because this group is flexible,
very adaptable to change, and comfortable with technology,
its members are powerful change agents. Xers like to
multitask, so it is important to keep this group challenged at
all times.

Even as patients, Xers are leaving their mark on
health care. Because this group tends to reject authority, as
patients they have turned to self-education via the Internet
as a replacement for physician-driven consultations and
education. As patients (consumers), they prefer the do-it-
yourself approach to health care and have learned how
to do their own research. So, nurses and other health care
professionals must learn new ways to communicate with
this very resourceful group. The use of various types of
educational materials is the best approach; they can then
read/listen to what most interests them and process the
information themselves (Washburn, 2000).

Millennials (Gen Yers)

This group is 78 million strong and was born between
1982 and approximately 2000 (Strauss & Howe, 1991).
The millennials grew up in the age of the Oklahoma
City bombing, Columbine shootings, and 9/11. The age
of terrorism has resulted in very protective parents and
family for this generation; think "Baby On Board" for this
group (Marston, 2010). They have seen mostly sad and
tragic stories on the news and have therefore adopted the
philosophy that you cannot be too careful, and they are
often taken care of by parents even well into adulthood
(Marston, 2011).

This group is confident, expressive, liberal, financially conservative, upbeat, and open to change. Its members are changing our political climate by showing the struggle between their open-mindedness and financial conservatism (Figure 2.4). They are the least religious generation in recent times. Of 2,020 millennials surveyed by Pew Research Center (2010), three out of four claim to be affiliated with a religion, which is lower than adults of other recent generations at the same age. They are also less likely to have served in the military; only 2% of millennial males are veterans, compared to 6% of Xer men, 13% of male boomers, and 24% of traditionalist men (Pew Research Center, 2010).

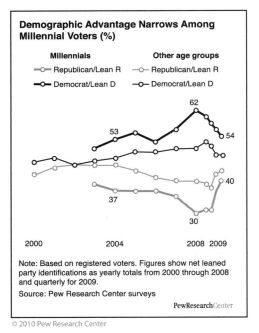

Demographic Advantage Narrows Among Millennial Voters (%)

Millennials
- —○— Republican/Lean R
- —●— Democrat/Lean D

Other age groups
- —○— Republican/Lean R
- —○— Democrat/Lean D

Note: Based on registered voters. Figures show net leaned party identifications as yearly totals from 2000 through 2008 and quarterly for 2009.
Source: Pew Research Center surveys

PewResearchCenter

© 2010 Pew Research Center

FIGURE 2.4

However, as individuals, millennials are extremely technology savvy; they are our first generation to grow up with computers. They are very optimistic, civic minded, sociable, strong networkers, sophisticated, and street smart, and they like to keep their options open (read: avoid commitment). They also see differences as strengths: Together we can get it done. Although this group is independent minded, its members like to make group decisions, and they especially like to travel in packs. Even though they have a group mentality and are comfortable in groups, millennials have a hard time sacrificing for the greater good. This is the only cohort that has grown up with a global economy. They are the most racially diverse and the best-educated generation to date.

WHY DO WE CALL THE LAST GROUP GENERATION Y?

Y should I get a job?
Y should I buy a car when I can borrow yours?
Y should I leave home and find my own place?
Y should I clean my room?
Y should I buy my own food?
–Author unknown

How do millennials affect the workplace? Remember that for much of this group, the start of their careers and their entry into the workforce has been delayed or altered by the Great Recession (Pew Research Center, 2010). This has caused much frustration. Even in nursing, we are unable to employ all the newly graduated nurses produced in the past few years.

Millennials like instant gratification and have an insatiable demand for feedback and recognition. Many desire to move up, even to executive-level positions, within a year. Impatience is one of this group's major characteristics. They find it frustrating when they do not get promoted quickly, and they are perfectly willing to quit and move to another organization if they think that will improve their chances of promotion. If you dig into your own turnover data, you will see this trend. These nurses misinterpret their more-senior nurse colleagues, who have been on the same unit for most (or all) of their careers and so have not taken advantage of opportunities. They cannot imagine that someone would have made the conscious decision to stay in one place within one organization on purpose.

Their level of commitment, for the most part, hinges on their perception of recognition within the organization. This often expresses itself when a staffing crunch occurs; they are less willing than some of their peers to pick up shifts or work extra hours.

> **NOTE**
>
> *From a nurse manager's perspective, it is important to know that millennials accept authority but desire immediate rewards and live in the present.*

Latest Generation

It appears as though the latest generation may have started sometime around 1995 to 2000, but this is difficult to determine at this point; the start of a new generation is typically determined retrospectively. There is also not a clear view of what this generation will be named—Generation Z, new millennials? It seems as though they could even be the Homeland Generation or the Great Recession Generation (Alsop, 2011). We are still watching and waiting as this group quietly takes its place among the generations. Raising two of these future employees myself, I think they are going to be more of a challenge to manage as employees than any of the other generations so far.

Workforce Differences

The unique and distinctive generational behaviors and traits exhibit themselves in the workplace and often show up as value differences related to the work environment, job/self-perception, work ethic, and so on (Table 2.2). There aren't necessarily good traits and bad traits, but it is essential to understand them and know how to motivate the workforce to attain its mission and goals.

TABLE 2.2
GENERATIONAL WORK VALUES

PERSONALITY TRAITS IN THE WORK ENVIRONMENT	
Traditionalists	Self-sacrificing for company goals.
Boomers	Team oriented, competitive, will do it their own way.
Xers	Self-reliant, meets job requirements.
Millennials	Multitasking, sharing, and networking.

PERCEPTION OF MY JOB	
Traditionalists	I am as successful as my job.
Boomers	My job defines me.
Xers	It's a job.
Millennials	I am what I do, not who I work for.

WORK ETHIC	
Traditionalists	Defined by clock (either on or off the clock).
	Strong work ethic.
Boomers	Visibility, workaholics, face time.
	Willing to work to get ahead.
Xers	Get the job done and move on.
	Striving for work-life balance.
Millennials	Use technology to make work more efficient to free up time.
	Want meaningful jobs and work-life balance.

continues >

TABLE 2.2, CONTINUED
GENERATIONAL WORK VALUES

WORK-RELATED ISSUES

Traditionalists	"Presenteeism" related to medical issues or depression.
	Absence related to medical concerns.
	Respect for diversity.
	Consequences of their lifestyle behaviors (for example, smoking and drinking).
Boomers	Tolerate the nontraditional work styles of Xers and millennials.
	Technology replacing human interaction.
	Sharing praise and rewards.
	Balancing work and family.
Xers	Career development.
	Conflict resolution.
	Office politics.
	Multigenerational team projects.
	Balancing work and family.
Millennials	Absence related to lifestyle decisions.
	Consequences of lifestyle or risk-taking behaviors.
	Respectful communication.
	Balancing work and social life.

WORK MOTIVATION

Traditionalists	Financial security.
Boomers	Self-fulfillment and meaning.
Xers	Meet financial need without too much demand on personal time.
Millennials	Fun and meaningful work.

Style

Traditionalists	Formal.
Boomers	Hierarchical.
Xers	Independent.
Millennials	Casual.

(Rich, 2008; Alsop, 2011; Hicks & Hicks, 1999; Karp, Fuller, & Sirias, 2002; Lancaster & Stillman, 2002; Meredith, 2002).

Job Satisfaction and Engagement

The literature suggests that employees born in 1945 or earlier appear to be more satisfied, whereas younger employees are often less satisfied, although this isn't always the case. As mentioned earlier, millennials can be very satisfied.

KEY POINT

A definite generation gap exists when it comes to employee satisfaction and engagement. Your job is to be aware of it and to work with all the generations to shrink the gap.

Workplace expectations have an influence on engagement and satisfaction. Younger generations, such as the Xers and millennials, have different expectations of the workplace than the previous generations. They look to the workplace to demonstrate that it values and recognizes the employees regularly for their contributions; when this doesn't occur as expected, they become disengaged and dissatisfied. However, although it is true that both millennials and Xers have a greater need to receive recognition, what they really desire is to be included in decisions and to engage in real-time communication with hospital leaders (Press Ganey Associates, 2012). These two generations were included in "family meetings" when young, so now they expect some input in the workplace; otherwise, they will not consider their voices to have been heard.

> **NOTE**
>
> *It is important for nurse managers to realize that as soon as employees become dissatisfied, they will move on to another unit or employer to find new happiness.*

For an organization to do well on employee engagement/satisfaction surveys, it is first important for nurse managers to understand the various needs and expectations that each generation has of its job and of its employer. Finally, the key to high engagement and satisfaction scores is that as a manager, you must realize that one size will *not* fit all. Each generation has special needs that have to be met to improve organizational satisfaction, engagement, and, ultimately, commitment. Involve the employees in the enhancements or changes that are made. This will reward them with the input they crave. In addition, don't be shy about reminding them that their voices have been heard.

> **NOTE**
>
> *It is essential to manage expectations and communicate clearly to avoid misunderstandings.*

Loyalty and Commitment

Why don't our Xer and millennial staff seem as loyal as our traditionalists and boomers? As children, the Xers lived through the recession of the mid-1970s and saw many parents get laid off from their jobs even after long-time employment with the same company. In return, this has planted a seed of caution that says, "Why should I stay when they can lay me off at any time?" Millennials have short attention spans for jobs, school, activities, and anything else. The roots of this can be traced back to toddler soccer, t-ball, flag football, or you-name-the-sport. If they didn't like it or it was too hard, parents often made it easy for them to change teams or sports or even quit altogether. This is an entire generation of young people who have been able to change or quit so easily that they have experience with multiple transitions but not with sticking it out.

The lesson that has been ingrained in this generation is that if it "isn't for you," you can ask for a change and expect to make it. I am not saying that this is right or wrong, just that it is different from previous generations. As an Xer, I can tell you that my parents taught me the very valuable lesson of sticking it out. If I joined something, I was sure to finish it, like it or not. This taught me the art of quiet suffering, but more important, it taught me to make good decisions about what to join. This translates into the work environment, as well: How many young nurses do you know who left their job within 12–18 months, or even left nursing altogether, because it wasn't what they wanted to do?

Adulthood
Five Milestones

The transition into adulthood has been different for each generation, causing family and social norms to change quite a bit over the past several decades. The millennials' approach to this transition is unique from any other, and they continue to write their own rules and to handle the traditional life milestones their own way. Sociologists have traditionally defined the transition to adulthood by marking the five milestones:

- Completing school
- Leaving home
- Becoming financially independent
- Getting married
- Having a child

In 1960, it was demonstrated that 77% of women and 65% of men reached these five milestones by the time they turned 30. However, in 2000, only 50% of women and 33% of men reached the five milestones by that same age. Is this just an American phenomena? It doesn't look like it. A Canadian study showed that in 2001, the typical Canadian 30-year-old completed the same number of milestones as a 25-year-old Canadian did in the early 1970s (Henig, 2010).

Emerging Adulthood

What may help explain some of this behavior is a new movement to define *emerging adulthood*, which is purportedly a new field of psychology. Emerging adulthood views the behavior of adults in their 20s as a distinct life stage of its own. Adults in this life stage have their own profile, which is characterized by identity exploration, self-focus, instability, and feeling "in between" (Henig, 2010).

The identification of a new life stage can be compared to more than a century ago, when social scientists evaluated social and economic changes of the time and designated *adolescence* as its own new life stage in 1904. The realization of this "new" life stage led the way to such innovations as junior high and middle schools to provide these sixth, seventh, and eighth graders what they needed educationally and developmentally. However, changes of this magnitude do not occur over night. It will take more study and more time before psychologists are, in fact, certain that emerging adulthood is its own life stage.

Boomeranging

The beginning of adulthood is markedly different from generation to generation. Traditionalists entering adulthood often had to get jobs to contribute to the family or to support their own new family, and many men served in World War II or the Korean War. Around the same age, boomers went to college or became involved in the Vietnam War. Xers started the trend of moving away from their parents' home either to college or otherwise out on their own. In an altogether different approach, one in eight millennials has left home just to return, or has "boomeranged," later to their parents' home (Pew Research Center, 2010). The most common reason cited is underemployment as a result of the recession. Returning home is difficult for both parents and the millennial, but because this generation tends to have very strong relationships with its parents and extended families, a lax attitude regarding the house rules is tolerated. This is so prevalent that it is no longer a sign of failure to move back in with Mom and Dad; it doesn't seem to bother boomerangers at all (Figure 2.5).

A national survey of 2,048 adults shows that 29% of adults ages 25 to 34 have found themselves in this situation in the past few years, and of those, 78% say that they are satisfied with these living arrangements. Of those who have returned to the nest, 25% report that the arrangements have negatively impacted their relationship with their parents, whereas 24% indicate that there has been a positive impact as a result, and almost half (48%) say it hasn't made any difference. This practice is more widespread than originally thought, as 61% of adults, ages 25 to 34, report that they know a friend who has moved back in with his or her parents, whereas 29% of parents surveyed indicated that a child of theirs has returned home to live (Pew Research Center, 2010).

Rising Share of Young Adults Living in Multi-Generational Households

% of adults ages 25-34 living in a multi-generational household

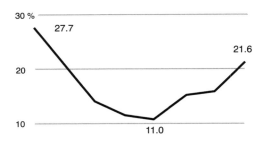

Source: Pew Research Center analysis of U.S. Decennial Census data, 1940-2000 and 2010 American Community Survey (IPUMS)

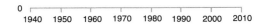

© 2010 Pew Research Center

FIGURE 2.5

To validate this trend, U.S. Census data indicate that the share of Americans residing in a multigenerational household is the highest it has been in decades, since the mid-1950s. The increase has mostly occurred in the past 5 years. This arrangement isn't always perceived as bad news; after all, the finances of a multigenerational household can benefit both adult children and their parents.

WHAT MAKES YOUR GENERATION UNIQUE?

Millennials
> Technology 24%
> Music/pop culture 11%
> Tolerant 7%
> Well educated 6%

(Pew Research Center, 2010)

This arrangement might remain steady for the near future. As a result of the economic environment over the past few years, the job outlook in general for young adults is less than favorable. The unemployment rate for our youngest workers (ages 18 to 24) has increased dramatically over 3 years, from 2007 to 2010, and has only recently begun to decrease slightly. Many new graduate nurses are unable to find nursing jobs or have to very aggressively compete with many other applicants over scarce entry-level nursing jobs for new graduates. This is sending a confusing message. As an industry, we begged for nursing schools to increase the workforce pipeline and produce more new graduates, and they responded. Now, many new grads are going unhired throughout the country. Clearly, this represents a challenge we must fix, and quickly, before the schools turn off the production spigot.

Marriage and Family

Millennials are reassessing their life priorities. What they indicate as a priority is not always the outcome we see. For example, even though 30% of millennials who responded to a Pew Research Center survey indicated that having a successful marriage is important, just over 20% of millennials are married, compared to more than 40% of their parents at the same age (Figure 2.6). Only 6 out of 10 millennials were raised in a two-parent household, which is lower than all the other generational cohorts at the same age (Pew Research Center, 2010). This percentage will likely drop even lower for the newest generation. There are many reasons for these changes, including increased educational opportunities, career options, and a changing society perspective about the acceptable age for marriage and family (CDC, 2012).

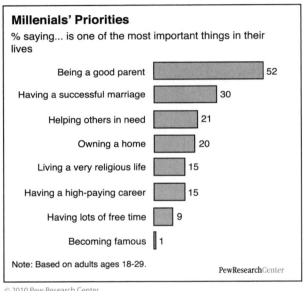

FIGURE 2.6

Millennials are starting a family later in life than did traditionalists, boomers, and even the Xers. This is one milestone that has clearly been pushed to later in life. Only 34% of millennials have children. The percentage of live births by mothers 35 years or older has increased from approximately 8% of all births in 1970 to approximately 12% of all births in 2000 (Figure 2.7). In addition, the average age of the mother at her first child's birth (Figure 2.8) has increased from approximately 21.5 years old in 1970 to nearly 24.5 years old in 2000 (CDC, 2012).

Another big change is that one-third of women who gave birth in 2006 were unmarried; this trend continues. Unmarried women giving birth is no longer socially unacceptable or taboo (Table 2.3). However, this practice differs markedly from the previous generations at the same age and is therefore hard for the older generations to understand (Pew Research Center, 2010). Know your staff and understand how these family differences may affect them. Do you know who your single parents are? Do you know who is recently married (or even divorced)? Know how to support staff through life-stage changes.

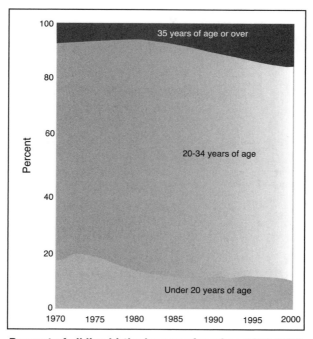

Percent of all live births by age of mother, 1970-2000

FIGURE 2.7
(Centers for Disease Control.)

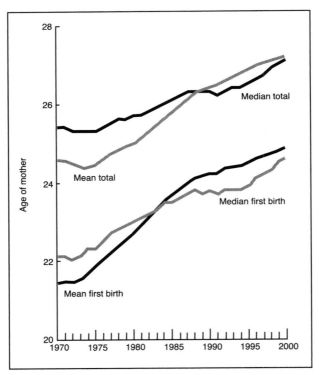

Mean and median age of mother by live birth order, 1970-2000

FIGURE 2.8

(Centers for Disease Control.)

TABLE 2.3

***MARRIAGE TRENDS IN MARRIAGE AND PARENTHOOD, BY
GENERATION*** (% saying this is a bad thing for society)

	Millennial	Gen X	Boomer	Silent
More single women deciding to have children	59	54	65	72
More gay couples raising children	32	36	48	55

	Millennial	Gen X	Boomer	Silent
More mothers of young children working outside the home	23	29	39	38
More people living together w/o getting married	22	31	44	58
More people of different race marrying each other	5	10	14	26

Note: "Good thing," "Doesn't make much difference," and "Don't know" responses not shown.

© 2010 Pew Research Center

Real-World Issues
Scheduling and 12-Hour Shifts

The schedules of the health care world vary wildly, but generally speaking our organizations run 24/7 operations, every day of the year, for years on end. Yet it continues to amaze me when nursing students or newly hired recently graduated nurses tell us that they can't work nights or weekends because of other commitments. Who do they think is going to work these shifts? Do we all just get to go home to bed and come back in the morning to check on the patients? Who is likely to be working weekends and holidays? The answer is often traditionalists and boomers, of course, unless the Xers and millennials need to raise money for something, in which case working (making money) is viewed as the lesser evil (borrowing money).

Xer and millennial nurses love the flexibility that 12-hour shifts represent. Three shifts per week means full-time employment with the benefits and perks that this includes. These nurses view this as very positive, because this kind of freedom allows them to pursue their favorite activities and hobbies at regular and predictable times, which is extremely important to this group. However, although this is viewed positively by Xer and millennial nurses, 12-hour shifts represent difficulty for many nurses in the upper ranges of the boomer and traditionalist generations. The length of these shifts means being on your feet for 12 hours straight, which is very tiring for many nurses. Often, our older nurses do not like this and look for opportunities to transfer to other departments where the shift length is more endurable for them.

To further compound this issue, a plethora of literature now indicates the patient safety challenges that 12-hour shifts represent. This places nurse managers and leaders in a very difficult position between patient safety and nurse satisfaction. Patient safety should always win in these situations, even knowing that the implications may mean nurses migrating to other areas. It is not uncommon for nurses to transfer to outpatient or ambulatory areas simply for the schedule change that this brings.

Flexibility is of utmost importance to Xers and millennials. Traditionalists and boomers are likely to deal with more-fixed schedules better without feeling such a heavy impact on their work-life balance; they have grown accustomed to it. Nurse managers need to discuss these issues with nursing students to align their expectations with reality before the students graduate from nursing school.

In a Staffing Pinch?

If your unit/department is short of staff and needs someone to stay late, come in early, or pick up a shift, how do you ask? Who will work? What can you expect? Although these are overly generalized answers, there is some humorous truth to them:

- The traditionalist nurse may say, "I have plans, but if you need me to, I can probably change them." (Read: I will help the team.)

- The boomer nurse might say, "I have plans, but if no one else can do it, I will do it." (Read: Someone has to take care of the patients.)

- The Xer nurse may say, "I have plans, but what's it worth to you?" (Read: For the right price, I will consider your offer.)

- The millennial is likely to say, "I just worked my shift, I have plans." (Read: Not my problem.)

Even though these are highly stereotypical responses, I have *heard* these responses and venture a bet that these scenarios are playing out regularly around the country. It is no secret that the older generations tend to be more committed and loyal than the younger generations. The lesson here is to know this in advance, anticipate these responses, and have a plan to make things work out.

Diversity

Nursing has been, is, and will continue to be a generationally diverse profession. Diversity in other areas is increasing, as well. We are seeing more age diversity, gender diversity, and ethnic diversity than ever before (Table 2.4, Table 2.5, and Figure 2.9). Due to the acceptance of interracial marriage in the 1970s and 1980s, the millennial generation is our most ethnically diverse generation thus far. However, in nursing, we continue to evolve through the diversity process. Although patients, nurses, and nursing students are becoming more ethnically and racially diverse, nursing school faculty is not. Increasing the diversity of faculty not only helps students be more successful in their own learning, but it also serves to create a school culture and produce nurses who are more like the communities that they serve. Advocacy, outreach, and recruitment of a more diverse faculty will remedy this over time (Tomer, 2012). Succession planning, in a way to promote diversity, will help your leadership team resemble your staff nurses.

TABLE 2.4
MEDIAN AGE OF REGISTERED NURSES

Survey Year	Median Age
2008	46
2004	46
2000	44
1996	42
1992	40
1988	38

Source: 1988-2008 National Sample Survey of Registered Nurses

TABLE 2.5
GENDER OF EMPLOYED REGISTERED NURSES, BY YEAR OF INITIAL REGISTERED NURSE LICENSE

	Licensed Before 2000		Licensed in 2000 or Later	
	Male	Female	Male	Female
Percentage of Employed Nurses	6.2	93.8	9.6	90.4
Median Age	49	50	35	31

(HRSA, 2010)

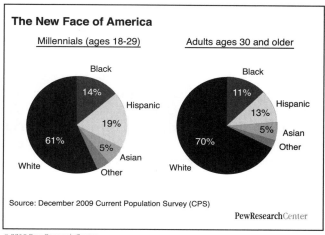

FIGURE 2.9

Summary

This chapter described how the four generations differ. As the newer generations age to where older generations are currently, will they then act in more similar ways to the older generations than they do now? It isn't looking like it. How do we get the generations to work better together considering the differences they experience while being raised, their different values, and ways of doing things. We can't wait for the various generations to align—it won't happen. For example, relying on adults to do things for them is something that this generation learned as toddlers. It was hardwired into their DNA; that isn't going to change.

Managing employees who are a generation apart in age can prove challenging, because different points of view often result in misunderstandings. However, it seems to be more difficult for younger managers to manage employees who are older than they are. To be successful, it is important to understand why each generation functions the way that it does. In addition, you must plan for interactions and responses so that you can clearly communicate expectations in a respectful manner so that all parties have a successful and positive outcome. Even difficult conversations should be delivered in a clear and respectful manner; although the content of the message might be uncomfortable, the receiver of the message will not be ruffled by any lack of respect.

Each generation has a distinct personality, style, and attitude, including perceptions about its work ethic, loyalty, communication style, and life goals. To be effective and run a successful department, a nurse manager needs to understand how to navigate through these differences and leverage them in a way that creates a functional and safe work environment.

References

Alsop, R. (2011). How the millennial generation is shaking up the workplace. *Workforce Management.*

Boychuk Duchscher, J. E., & Cowin, L. (2004). Multigenerational nurses in the workplace. *Journal of Nursing Administration, 34*(11), 493–501.

Bureau of Labor Statistics (BLS). (2012). Retrieved from http://www.bls.gov/news.release/ecopro.t01.htm

Centers for Disease Control (CDC). (2012). Retrieved from http://www.cdc.gov/nchs/births.htm

Henig, R. M. (2010). What is it about 20-somethings? *New York Times Magazine*. Retrieved from http://www.nytimes.com/2010/08/22/magazine/22Adulthood-t.html?pagewanted=all

Hicks, R., & Hicks, K. (1999). *Boomers, X'ers, and other strangers*. Wheaton, MA. Tyndale House Publishers.

Health Resources and Services Administration (HRSA). (2012). Retrieved from http://www.hrsa.gov/about/news/pressreleases/2010/100922nursingworkforce.html

Karp, H., Fuller, C., and Sirias, D. (2002). Bridging the boomer-X'er gap: Creating authentic teams for high performance at work. Palo Alto, CA. Davies-Black Publishing.

Lancaster, L., & Stillman D. (2002). *When generations collide*. New York, NY. Harper Business.

Marshburn, D. & Scott, E. (2009). *New nurses are not all alike: Meeting the diverse transition needs of newly licensed nurses*. Presentation, March 10, 2009.

Marston, C. (2010). *Generational insights*. Mobile, AL: Generational Insights.

Marston, C. (2011). *How to train millennials*. Mobile, AL: Generational Insights.

Meredith, G. S. (2002). *Managing by defining moments*. New York, NY. Wiley.

Pew Research Center. (2010). *Pew social & demographic trends*. Pew Charitable Trust.

Press Ganey Associates. (2012). Engaging the youngest workers on your team. Retrieved from http://www.pressganey.com/newsLanding/10-07-20/Engaging_the_youngest_workers_on_your_team.aspx#

Rich, P. (2008). Engaging the multi-generational workforce. *HR Management*. Retrieved from http://www.hrmreport.com/article/Engaging-the-Multi-generational-Workforce/

Satran, P. (2009). *How not to act old*. New York: HarperCollins Publishers.

Smola, K., & Sutton, C. (2002). Generational differences: Revisiting generational work values for the new millenium. *Journal of Organizational Behavior*, *23*, 363–382.

Stanley, D. (2010). Multigenerational workforce issues and their implications for leadership in nursing. *Journal of Nursing Management, 18,* 846–852.

Strauss, W., & Howe, N. (1991). *Generations.* New York: William Morrow & Company.

Tomer, J. (2012). Welcome to the future: The next generation of minority nurses. *Minority Nurse,* 23–27.

Washburn, E. (2000). Are you ready for Generation X? *Physician Executive, 26*(2), 51–57.

Wolburg, J., & Pokrywczynski, J. (2001, September-October). A psychographic analysis of Generation Y college students. *Journal of Advertising Research, 41*(5), 33–52.

3

Communication and Self-Expression

If I were given the opportunity to present a gift to the next generation, it would be the ability for each individual to learn to laugh at himself.

–Charles M. Schultz

Communication could not possibly play a more important role in patient safety and patient care. The data from unfortunate events show us how poor communication or even miscommunication leads to errors and mishaps. However, as nurse managers, we don't receive training on the best way to communicate or how to get the message out to the right audience (and ensure that it is interpreted as intended). In addition to our traditional forms of communication in nursing, such as one-on-one communication, staff meetings, e-mails, and memos, newer forms of communication continue to evolve. These include texting, blogs, websites, and social media postings. Expecting your generationally diverse staff to all use the same method of communication is wishful thinking (and will result in a failure to get the word out as you intend if you rely on such an expectation). In today's environment, nurse managers need to consider mixed modes of communication, such as staff meetings with e-mails, texts, or even website postings of the agendas and summaries. As a manager, your job is to get the message out effectively to as many of the intended audience as possible.

This chapter covers:

- Generational differences in communication patterns and styles

- The impact of social media

- Generational differences in appearance and self-expression

Communication Differences

Believe it or not, each generation has its own communication patterns and preferences. For example, traditionalists prefer face-to-face communication, via staff meetings or hallway conversations, as the means to receive information. They perceive these means as ways to build trust and consider them the most effective ways to communicate. E-mail and texting are not reliably effective modes of communication for this group.

Baby boomers are somewhat averse to technology, with older boomers tending to be digitally naïve. They often ask their children or grandchildren to program phones and computers, and they have given in to the fact that technology is an ever-increasing part of patient care (Beard, 2010). The typical boomer communication style includes open, direct, and less-formal (than traditionalist) dialogue. This group tends to prefer face-to-face group meetings and even telephone calls, because these communication methods allow for two-way dialogue.

Xers tend to prefer e-mail to phone calls, but they have really caught on to texting. Direct, get-to-the-point communication is best for this group. Xers prefer the use of technology over lengthy discussions, and in their opinion, this is most efficiently accomplished via e-mail. They want to avoid "wasting" the time required to have a discussion when all they really want know is "What's the bottom line?" Summaries, bullet points, and metrics that show progress in relation to goals are helpful for this group. Xers prefer a work culture with open channels of communication and one that allows them to freely share their opinions. To many, Xers often seem impatient and demanding of an overabundance of information. But remember, this is the first generation to have been raised from birth with television sets, so they are used to constant input and sound-bites and crave streaming, real-time information. Cutting off communication or limiting information is a sure way to alienate an Xer.

Overall, millennials prefer fragmented, abbreviated, and frequent communication. They are perceived to be rude, direct, and blunt and are even known for their frequent interruptions. In reality, they just want to be heard and want to be part of the conversation. Millennials value work environments that allow them to express themselves, offer their opinions, and learn from colleagues. They also value environments where they can freely share ideas via electronic means as well as in person.

As a nurse manager, the key takeaway is to facilitate open and honest communication through a variety of modalities.

Millennials have had cell phones, computers, and the Internet since birth and think that the norm is instant gratification or instant knowledge as it unveils itself through the use of technology (Beard, 2010). Cell phones are like an electronic tether for this group, a lifeline. Cell phones allow for daily regular communication with friends and family. Millennials prefer communicating via texts, blogs, microblogs (Twitter), or websites to using face-to-face communication and find gratification in responding instantly (Beard, 2010). Paradoxically, this generation prefers group meetings to lengthy e-mails and memos. Some millennials see e-mail as archaic and for dinosaurs or "old" people; in their mind, composing an e-mail takes way too long.

Millennials have taken to texting like fish to water, hence the prolific use of texting to communicate among this group. It is not uncommon to see a group of millennials sitting together but texting each other. They don't find this unusual at all; instead, they find it rather normal. The upside is a much faster way to communicate, the downside is that the "language" of texting, such as LOL (laughing out loud) or RME (rolling my eyes), has even crept into their written work and projects. The problem isn't that you have to help them correct the work; the problem is often that they don't see it as wrong.

The Impact of Different Communication Styles

Undoubtedly, four different communication styles concurrently in the workplace have an impact. For example, you'll find in the workplace different speaking styles, the use of vernacular, and even variations in response times. Because millennials were raised in a more casual environment than were the other generations, some communication challenges arise. For instance, their parents reared them more as friends than as children and often allowed them to call older people (neighbors/family friends) by their first names, something that was mostly unacceptable before this generation. So, millennials often refer to their parent's friends or older neighbors by their first names instead of using Mr. or Mrs. and find it difficult to ascertain when this behavior is acceptable and when it is not. Millennials are perfectly comfortable calling their much older patients Bob or Marilyn rather than Mr. Clipper or Mrs. Clipper. The millennial intends no disrespect, but traditionalist patients often interpret it as such. In contrast, traditionalists were reared in a much more formal and hierarchical manner. They had to refer to adults and people of influence (teachers, policemen, firemen, religious leaders, and so on) by their formal titles, using Mr. and Mrs. and even "yes ma'am" and "no sir." Therefore, the casual nature of millennial communication, and to a lesser degree Xer communication, confounds them. They don't understand it, and they don't like it.

Managing employees who are a generation or more apart from yourself can be a challenge, because you will sometimes feel like you're not even speaking the same language as they are speaking. The meanings of words and expressions do change over time. For example, my high-school-age son went into hysterics when I told him I was "hooking up" with some friends for dinner. He then explained to me the current meaning of that term; I was mortified. How was I to know that the meaning had changed from something that I was familiar with to something that was now X-rated?

NOTE

As a nurse manager, try to be attuned to current phrases and word usage. You cannot reasonably know the meaning of all slang for four generations, so just try to be a fast learner and be ready to laugh at yourself from time to time.

TABLE 3.1
CROSS-GENERATIONAL COMMUNICATION

Traditionalist and Boomers	Xers and Millennials
We're invincible as a team.	I work best alone.
Highly value participation and consensus.	Do not need to participate, attend meetings, or hear others' opinions.
Value what others think.	Care very little about what others think.
I want, I think, I'd like....	I need....
Softened communication style.	Short, abrupt, and casual speech.
Recognition is important.	Recognition isn't important; I know what kind of job I'm doing.

Answering Questions

You might not have realized this, but there are even generational differences in the allowable *response time* following a question. As a nurse manager, you need to understand how something even as subtle as response time has been predetermined by each generation and how it impacts communication with employees. Response time is generally based on each generation's collective life experiences and has formed into a norm for them.

For example, if a traditionalist nurse asks you a question, she (very few men in this group) is going to wait patiently for approximately 7 to 10 days for your answer. This group grew up in a time when a question often took the form of a letter; the recipient of the letter had to take time to answer it and send a return letter in response. So to some degree, the answer was tied to the response time of the post office.

When boomer nurses ask a question, they will wait patiently for about a day or two. When they were growing up, questions were asked with a phone call. After the call was placed, someone of authority had to determine the answer before a return call that provided the response could be made.

In this same scenario, if Xer nurses ask a question, they will wait patiently for approximately the length of a shift. After all, based on their life experience, that represents the amount of time that it *should* take a manager to make a decision, track down someone who can approve it or who knows the answer, and communicate it back to the person inquiring.

When millennials ask a question, their patience for an answer is approximately 5 minutes, because that is approximately how long it would take them to find the answer on the Internet. Anything longer than that is likely to frustrate them, as it seems like you are stalling or cannot provide an answer.

Now you understand why the generations have different expectations regarding something as simple as response time to a question.

Providing Feedback

People often find feedback difficult, both in terms of giving it and receiving it. As with many things discussed thus far, nurse managers want to account for generation differences when they provide feedback to staff. Traditionalists prefer feedback to be given in private and are often prepared for the worst. They will work hard to correct any deficiencies brought to their attention.

Boomers take constructive feedback as very personal information and work hard to make improvements. Ideally, you need to do this as part of a private, one-on-one discussion and never in front of anyone else. When it comes to recognition, however, this group responds very favorably to recognition provided in group settings (Kramer, 2010).

Xers, in contrast, take feedback as very personal and critical. Sometimes they even find it difficult to "hear" your key message through the discussion, because they may focus on one or two phrases and overinterpret those as the entire message. *Sandwiching* the feedback is a good option with this group. For example, provide Xers with something positive—something constructive—something positive. This group likes recognition but can take it or leave it. Really, they just want to be thanked for their contribution, no matter how small.

Millennials have a hard time receiving constructive feedback, because most of their lives they have had people telling them that whatever they are working on is good. They do like feedback, though, and see it as a course corrector; it helps them change the way that they do things to do even better. They like to receive feedback often and in small bite-size pieces. For example, "You did a good job with that fresh post-op admit. Next time you might think about doing this or that differently, but good job." Don't wait until you have a few things to provide feedback on; otherwise, they feel attacked. Remember, we have showcased their art and schoolwork on our refrigerator galleries for many years. When providing recognition, remember that they like to be the center of attention and be recognized in front of their peers. After all, for this generation, we made a big deal of giving even the losing team trophies. The key takeaway here is that this group likes to feel special.

Communication Modalities

As you know, there are different ways that communication can occur, including verbal communication, nonverbal communication and written communication. If you were to drill down into each of these types of communication, you would also have several other more detailed types of communication. For example, verbal communication may occur in person, over the phone (or videophone), or via recorded message, to name a few. Nonverbal communication occurs through the signals we send by out expressions and gestures, while written communication may occur through books, letters, e-mails, text messages, and even through social media. We will discuss the impact of various types of communication on each generation.

Social Media

Social media is rapidly changing the way we communicate, share information, and even work. It is just one part of the information superhighway that is quickly becoming the key to staying connected with friends and family and is available at your fingertips. These platforms transform our communication and ability to share information. This is true not only of our interactions with our friends and family but also with health care providers. However, the social media-rich environment in which we live raises certain issues. You might be unsurprised to learn that nearly 75% of millennials have profiles on social networking sites and one in five has even posted a video of him- or herself online (Figure 3.1). One positive note here is that most millennials actually have privacy settings secure enough to protect their social networking profiles (Pew Research Center, 2012).

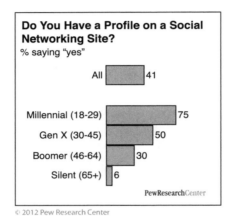

© 2012 Pew Research Center

FIGURE 3.1

Social media and even the Internet in general raise new concerns over privacy, including privacy of patients, colleagues, physicians, and even personal privacy. This concern applies especially to millennials. For this group's members, the lines of privacy are blurred in terms of where privacy starts and their right to free speech ends. I occasionally speak to senior nursing students about transitioning into the real world, and many nursing students are surprised that employers actually review Facebook pages. The retort that I typically hear from students is this: "That's my private page, and it shouldn't be used that way." I reply, "I am able to access it, and I am not your real-life friend, so it clearly isn't private." Using good judgment when posting comments and photos on social media sites is extremely important. This is not just true of job seekers either.

Patient privacy is more of a concern now than ever. As I talk to nurse executives around the country, it is no longer rare to learn of potential privacy violations by staff members who happened to see a colleague's inappropriate posting in the social media world. Many organizations have social media guidelines (or even a policy). Staff members need to feel free to ask questions openly and honestly about the policies and practices to ensure that they understand your expectations. The same goes for blogging or microblogging (Twitter).

NOTE

Make sure that all of your staff, especially your Xer and millennial staff, understand their obligations to protect patient privacy and that violations will not be tolerated.

Cell Phones

The millennials are the only generation that has had exposure to cell phones and the Internet from birth. This cohort has been reared on technological advances that traditionalists and even most boomers would have found inconceivable in their early lives. For millennials, the cell phone has become the electronic umbilical cord; they are never far from it, and it is a crisis if it is lost or nonfunctional. Cell phones are no longer just a phone but rather a true lifeline. Believe it or not, 83% of millennials surveyed by the Pew Research Center (2012) indicated that they sleep with their cell phones (Figure 3.2). Smart phones are indispensable. They are communication devices, provide GPS capability, and have more than 100,000 "apps" to help us live our lives each day (and apparently many of us can't live without them).

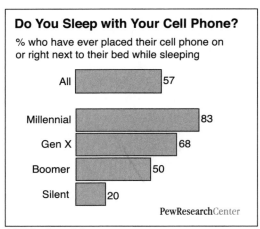

FIGURE 3.2

Technology continues to increase its presence in our lives and is here to stay, allowing all generations to become more efficient with their time. It is no surprise that the owners of cell phones are predominantly millennials (Figure 3.3). Xers are a close second in their reliance on technology, have a very tech-savvy nature, and have quickly adapted in this fast-paced and information-rich society in which we live.

% of Adults by Generation Who Own Each Device

	Millennials	Xers	Boomers	Traditionalists	All Adults (18+)
Cell phone	95	92	85	58	85
Desktop computer	57	69	65	38	59
Laptop computer	70	61	46	20	52
iPod/MP3 player	74	56	34	9	47

	Millennials	Xers	Boomers	Traditionalists	All Adults (18+)
e-Book reader	5	5	5	4	5
Tablet device	5	5	4	1	4
None of these	1	3	8	31	9

Information derived from the Pew Research Center's Internet & American Life Project, 2010

Pew Research Center's Internet & American Life Project, 2010. Retrieved from www. pewinternet.org/Reports/2011/Generations-and-gadgets/Overview.aspx. Accessed on October 10, 2012.

© 2012 Pew Research Center

FIGURE 3.3

Self-Expression

Nurses and nursing students do not have the same personal backgrounds that they used to. It is not uncommon today to evaluate a pool of potential nursing students that contains at least one applicant who has had a previous MIP (minor in possession) charge. Is this a new phenomenon? Probably not. But what is new is that either more young people are getting caught or it is happening more than it used to. Determining whether to admit a potential nursing student with an MIP was not part of the evaluation process even just a few years ago. This is just one of the changes evident in the younger generations.

In addition to not having the squeaky clean backgrounds that they used to, new nurses and nursing students often do not have the same look or appearance that they have traditionally had. Individuality and self-expression is very important to millennials, as reflected in tattoos, vivid hair colors, and piercings. However, in a health care setting, these appear unprofessional and even out of place. Traditionalist and boomer managers often wrinkle their noses in distaste as millennials show up to nursing school clinical rotations and job interviews proudly displaying their tattoos and blue hair.

A 2010 study (Pew Research Center) indicated that 38% of millennials have a tattoo. Among Xers, 32% percent are inked, whereas only 15% percent of boomers have a tattoo. Employers often require that employees cover visible tattoos with long sleeves or even an adhesive bandage, so as to not "affect" their patient's perception of their care. Tattoos are intended to be merely self-expression and may include hopes, dreams, loved ones, and even memorable places traveled. However, to boomer or traditionalist patients or coworkers, the stereotype of tattoos is that they are something that gang members, former prisoners, or other undesirables have (not something well-educated, highly competent health care staff has). Tattoos clearly show a generation gap. Certainly, there is a lack of understanding or even willingness by all sides to understand body art as self-expression.

WHAT MAKES YOUR GENERATION UNIQUE?

Xers
    Technology 12%
    Work ethic 11%
    Conservative 7%
    Smarter 6%
    Respectful 5%
    Values 10%

© 2010 Pew Research Center

Even though society finds tattoos less shocking than in earlier times, employers have not warmed up to them in health care. Therefore, the compliance struggle continues: As long as we continue to see tattoos among our nurses, we will continue to have enforcement challenges. Over time, as managers and nurses continue to age and move into the same generation as their patients, body art will likely be viewed in a less negative light. It is likely at that time the talk will turn from "no visible" tattoos permitted to which tattoos are acceptable and thus will be tolerated (Pyrillis, 2010).

> **NOTE**
>
> *The role of the nurse manager is to help Xer and millennial nurses understand the rationale for why tattoos need to be covered, or piercings removed, in the workplace and then consistently monitor the expectation.*

Piercings highlight an even larger generation gap. In the same study, nearly 25% of millennials surveyed have a piercing other than an on their earlobes. This compares to 9% of Xers and only 1% of boomers (Pew Research Center, 2010). In a study regarding piercings among health care providers, patients indicated that female caregivers (in general) who had facial piercings were perceived as less professional, confident, efficient, and approachable than nonpierced females (Westerfield, 2012). One person's art form is another person's form of self-mutilation. Xers and millennials contest that they are only expressing themselves and feel that people of older generations are overinterpreting the point. Body art is now a fashion statement and an acceptable art form, and to Xers and millennials, it does not conjure up the negative stigma that it does for boomers and traditionalists. It is what it is.

> **NOTE**
>
> *Nurse managers need to help traditionalists and boomers understand that they cannot use their value sets to judge their younger colleagues.*

Summary

Each generation has its own style of communication, acceptable fashion, patterns of speech, vocabulary, haircuts—almost anything, really. These differences are not necessarily good or bad, but rather the differences that set each generation apart. Each generation brings something new and unique to clearly establish its place in history. As nurse managers, it is important to understand the rationale or meaning behind the differences so that you can help all the generations better understand each other. It is easy to place our values on someone else, but that is not the right thing to do, especially if the other person's values derive from a different "place" than ours.

> **NOTE**
>
> *Communication is the most important piece of the puzzle in health care. We need to know how to communicate with each other and how to make sure we get the message across so that we provide the safest and best quality care possible.*

This chapter covered:

- Generational differences in communication patterns and styles
- The impact of social media
- Generational differences in appearance and self-expression

Leading staff of different backgrounds and generations takes creative and open-minded nurse managers. Each group has its own set of values that guides its philosophy and how it communicates. Having an understanding and awareness of the differences is a good place for nurse managers to operate from to build a cohesive team. The overall goal is teamwork and harmony, not standardization of communication styles.

References

Beard, K. (2010). Generational divide. *Advance for Nurses*, 12–13.

Kramer, L. W. (2010). Generational diversity. *Dimensions of Critical Care Nursing, 29*(3), 125–128.

Pew Internet Research. (2012). Cell phone ownership & trends. Retrieved from http://pewinternet.org/Presentations/2011/Apr/ FTC-Debt-Collection-Workshop-Cell-Phone-Trends.aspx

Pew Research Center. (2010). *Pew social & demographic trends.* Pew Charitable Trust. Retrieved from http:\\pewresearch.org\ pubs\1501\millennials-new-survey-generational-personality-upbeat-open-new-ideas-technology-bound

Pyrillis, R. (2010). Body of work. *Workforce Management*, 21–28.

Westerfield, H. S. (2012). Patients' perceptions of patient care providers with tattoos and/or body piercings. *Journal of Nursing Administration, 42*(3), 160–164.

4

Transition, Performance Management, and Succession Planning

We have the power to make this the best generation of
mankind in the history of the world—or to make it the last.
–*John Fitzgerald Kennedy*

Working with nurses across all four generations is
challenging, because each generational group has its
own way of doing things. When it comes to how nurses
are oriented to their new position or how you manage a
nurse's performance, many variables affect how you can
influence their behaviors. Another area strongly influenced

by generational differences is succession planning; this too requires adjustments to be made to accommodate for generational nuances. Learning key tactics and strategies to improve onboarding new staff, performance management, and career advancement will help you improve the outcomes of your team and ultimately allow your unit to provide better patient care, all providing increased job satisfaction for you, the nurse manager.

This chapter covers:

- The transition process, the use of preceptors, and the socialization of new staff

- Performance management advice related to the various generations

- The influence of generational differences on succession-planning and career-advancement practices

Transition to Practice

For young nurses, the transition to practice is difficult. It has been compared to moving to a foreign country and learning an unfamiliar language and culture (Keller, Meekins, & Summers, 2006). This is especially true when compounded by the generational differences of preceptors and coworkers. This degree of transition is anxiety producing and can even cause new graduates to question their choice of career/position. Studies have found that negative perceptions by the newly graduated nurse in the first 60 to 90 days of employment often lead to turnover within the first year (Wisotzkey, 2011). This is why it is so important to provide a smooth transition and a good orientation for these young nurses.

Orientation

Orientation differs from transition in that transition is a process whereby the new graduate nurse is learning about the profession, assimilating knowledge, and learning to function in his or her new role. Orientation more or less represents a key part of the new graduate nurse's transition into the organization and is specific to his or her new role and department. The orientation process helps to frame an organization's "way of doing things." These guardrails are necessary for all new nurse hires, even experienced nurses, but are especially important to new graduate nurses. As we now know, both orientation, to a new job and/or organization, and transition are equally anxiety producing. By identifying the right new hires, matching these new nurses with talented preceptors, and building in the appropriate support systems, we can minimize the negative perceptions and anxiety among new nurses and thus reduce the negative impact on first-year nurse retention.

Although orientation and transition differences exist for each of the generations upon starting a new job, specific concerns relate to millennials. For new millennial nurses, improved communication and social connections during the transition and orientation phase could decrease stress, which is at its peak after the first 3 to 6 months (Lee, Lin, & Yeh, 2009). This stress might arise because, among other things, millennials have been raised to be free spirits and to do whatever they want, at whatever time they want to do it. However, nursing is very structured, with patients requiring treatments and medications at specific times. In addition, many of the millennials are holding their first full-time job (read: responsibility).

> **NOTE**
>
> *Nurse managers should know that the highest first-year newly graduated nurse retention rates correspond directly with a 3-to-6-month orientation coupled with a preceptor model.*

These younger nurses require not only an orientation to the new job, environment, and personnel but also a carefully planned transition from their role as nursing student to an independent, professional nurse. For this to happen seamlessly, orientation should be tailored to meet the needs of each new nurse. The transition phase should include the following (Cowin & Hengstberger-Sims, 2006):

- Gradual increase of workload
- Minimal use of mentors/preceptors
- Close monitoring by the preceptor

This formalized transfer of responsibility serves as their welcome to the real world.

Unsurprisingly, a well-planned and well-executed orientation is also one of the key drivers of patient safety. If you need to be convinced about how important the orientation of inexperienced, new nurses is to safety, here is some data for you. The ineffective orientation of newly graduated nurses contributes to adverse events, as demonstrated in a study by the Joint Commission (2004) that showed of 1,690 adverse events over a 5-year period, 24% of these related to training of staff and to human error. To focus in on this issue, the inadequate training of new employees attributed to 58% of these errors (Joint Commission, 2004; Thompson, 2004).

In another example, a study of 1,000 newly graduated nurses showed that more than 20% of them had been involved in errors related to patient falls (Kenward & Zhong, 2006). In addition, we know that patient care from nurses with less experience contributes to an increase in wound infections and the mortality associated with these infections (Morrow, 2009). Highlighting the impact of newly graduated nurses on nursing practice, another study found that by matching RN characteristics with 2006 data from the National Database of Nursing Quality Indicators (NDNQI), each additional year of nursing experience decreases the fall rate by 1% (Dunton, Gajewski, Klaus, & Pierson, 2007).

NOTE

In order to be effective, orientation should be tailored to meet the needs of the individual graduate nurse.

Orienting nurses of the different generations requires generational-specific tactics and interventions (Table 4.1).

TABLE 4.1
ORIENTATION TIPS

Traditionalists	Take time to explain. Share the organization's story. Bring them into the goals of the group. Tell how they can contribute.
Boomers	Emphasize goals and challenges. Show them the opportunities.
Xers	Show technology. Allow time for exploring. Tell them who's who and how to locate resources. Repeat the work-life balance message over and over. Deemphasize workplace politics.
Millennials	Be clear about expectations. Show opportunities. Emphasize quality. Offer a lot of support.

(ICHRN, 2009)

Socialization

The more time the preceptors spend acclimating new team members to their new team, the better the transition process works for everyone. The goal of effective socialization is for the newly graduated nurse to successfully move through the continuum of reality shock to workplace adjustment. Successful completion of this process imparts a sense of pride, camaraderie, and accomplishment, which makes newly graduated nurses feel commitment toward their new team. As we know, commitment and job satisfaction are two of the foundational building blocks needed to build a climate of retention (Scott, Keehner Engelke, & Swanson, 2008).

Socialization is very important, because the newly graduated nurses do not have the life experience to know even the most simple of norms, such as what to bring for their meal, where to eat, how to dress, how to locate resources, where to park, where the break room/lockers are, and the chain of command. All of this must be taught as part of the socialization process. New team members welcomed by the existing staff each day are more likely to feel like part of the team, be satisfied in their new surroundings, and therefore stay on their unit.

In nursing, however, we have a terrible habit of eating our young. It is the twisted practice of treating new hires like we were (or think we were) treated. In fact, this is bullying in the workplace; we now know this as *incivility in the workplace*. There is no place for this in nursing. As a nurse manager, it is your job to keep your eyes and ears, or designated eyes and ears, open and on the lookout for this kind of behavior. If you see it or hear about it, deal with it immediately. Nurse managers need to provide a professional practice environment where everyone is respected, feels comfortable, and can share their opinions. Remember, multiple studies demonstrate that nurses with higher satisfaction have a stronger intention to stay, and such retention is vital to running a successful department.

> **TIP**
>
> *Don't bring treats without a reason. Acting like the department mommy only shows that you are, in fact, older than they are (Satran, 2009).*

Preceptors

As we have discussed, orientation is a key part of the new graduate nurse's acclimation to the organization. Orientation programs that facilitate the smooth transition from nursing student to newly graduated nurse have shown promise in reducing first-year newly graduated nurse turnover (Wisotzkey, 2011). The use of a preceptor-based orientation program is intended to prepare new graduate nurses to optimize their transition to practice in a supportive environment.

Use of Preceptors

As you know, preceptors are an integral part of the orientation process. How smoothly the orientation process proceeds depends to a large degree on the strength of the preceptors; they can, after all, ensure a smooth entry into nursing and help mitigate the transition shock of the newly graduated nurse. For the transition experience to prove successful, however, preceptors need training on how to facilitate this process.

Selecting Preceptors

Nurse manager identification and support of preceptors is essential. You can make improvements to your orientation process and your first-year nurse retention just by selecting the right nurses to be preceptors. Ideally, preceptors should be nurses across all generations who are middle to high performers, have strong clinical and communication skills, and are unit/department champions. This is not the role for your complainers or the nurses who fit the "he/she is a good nurse but..." description. This role should be reserved for those nurses whom you want to clone. Strong preceptors are solid role models for the newly graduated nurses to emulate. By learning and imitating their preceptors, newly graduated nurses can develop clinical skills and critical thinking patterns and acclimate to their new work environment (Lee et al., 2009).

Matching Preceptors With New Hires

The art of matching preceptors with their preceptee is important, because nothing is more important than fit. Some conflicts typically result when some of the generations are paired. For example, because of traditionalists' and boomers' nurturing nature, they do well as preceptors for millennials. However, Xers are often at odds with millennials in a preceptor relationship. Placing Xers with mentors is a challenge. Xers can be difficult to place with traditionalists, because Xers view them as hovering too much. Xers sometimes have a difficult time when paired with boomers, too, because Xers view the boomers as overly structured and process oriented. This makes it a challenge to pair Xers with a preceptor in general, unless it is with another Xer.

Nothing is impossible, though. It often comes down to the individuals/personalities involved making the best fit possible. Each generation typically does well with a preceptor of the same generation. The fit that you are looking for has to do with personality, attitude, and even hobbies or interests. As long as the preceptors also understand some of the generational nuances and can respond accordingly, the match should prove successful. Your job as a nurse manager is to match preceptees with the best preceptor possible to ensure success for both parties and then to regularly monitor the transition.

Preceptor Training

Because of the highly influential role preceptors play for newly graduated nurses, they require training and support to be high performers and to make the newly graduated nurses successful in their transition. Improving the effectiveness of preceptors is likely to be one of the enhancements that contribute most positively to first-year nurse retention. Well-prepared preceptors "contribute in no small measure to improving the job satisfaction and chances of retention of new graduates in a supportive clinical environment" (Henderson, Fox & Malko-Nyhan, 2006). A preceptor development program, including time for preceptor training and ongoing preceptor competency development, is a strong tool for organizations pursuing improved retention of first-year newly graduated nurses.

Preceptor development programs are defined as structured development programs focused on providing preceptors with the knowledge and tools to facilitate the transition of the new hires. The goal of these programs is to strengthen the preceptor's own skills and competencies as a means to improve the overall orientation and transition experience of the newly graduated nurse. To accomplish a successful transition, preceptors should be trained to understand generational differences in communication and learning styles. The preceptor's ability to understand generational differences is essential to employing strategies to successfully orient new graduate nurses. Tactics to minimize generational conflict and improve integration of newly graduated nurses not only helps the new nurse but also improves the effectiveness of the preceptor.

PRECEPTOR TACTICS

Ensure that preceptors receive annual preceptor refresher training.

Make sure that preceptors are still high or middle performers.

Work hard at the personality and communication-style pair matching.

Give preceptors a break from precepting when they request it.

In addition to incorporating generational differences into preceptor training, the actual design of the preceptor program should also accommodate generational differences. Preceptors are from every generation, and their development must be individualized for the most favorable results. Retention of high-quality preceptors is important to the development and retention of future new graduate nurses.

PRECEPTOR TRAINING GOALS

Educate preceptors to improve the orientation outcomes of new graduate nurses.

Decrease first year new graduate nurse turnover.

Improve perceptions of new graduate nurse orientation and onboarding processes.

In addition to generational differences, a structured preceptor development program should include training content to address as many of the newly graduated nurse concerns as possible, such as role transition, conflict resolution, delegation, and critical thinking skills.

Nurse managers should provide preceptor development often enough to keep pace with needs, making sure to have enough preceptors on all shifts to allow every new hire access to a well-trained preceptor. By doing so, you gain preceptor "bench strength," which then allows you to match preceptors appropriately with newly graduated nurses or new hires to ensure an optimal fit.

PRECEPTOR TRAINING TOPICS

Adult Learning & Teaching Principles
Novice to Expert Continuum
Generational Differences in Learning
Preceptor Roles & Responsibilities
Validating Competency
Providing Constructive Feedback & Coaching
Principles of Evaluation
Methods of Evaluation
Electronic Resources for Preceptors

You want to try to make preceptor training as cost-effective as possible, so stick to must-have topics. Ideally, you should leverage the content and instructors to benefit the organization, not just one department. This makes the return on investment even better and strengthens the business case for preceptor training. You can also use a variety of educational formats to cost-effectively engage each generation. Educational content offered online allows for self-paced learning and lessens the classroom/instructor investment necessary. The investment in preceptor preparation demonstrates commitment and support to the newly graduated nurses and improves the likelihood that they will stay with your organization. Preceptor training is also a win for the preceptors.

THE HOSPITAL DISCONNECT AMONG MILLENNIALS	
Typical Hospital Culture	**Millennials**
Hierarchical	Workplace flexibility
24/7 operations	Flexible schedules, active social lives
Fixed work hours	Multitaskers
Face-to-face communication	Texting and cell phones
Separation of work from personal life	Integration of work and personal life
Limited career mobility	Multiple jobs
Education doesn't necessarily facilitate mobility	Self-directed
Highly regulated	

(AHA, 2010)

Performance

Each generation has different perceptions, definitions, and expectations related to performance and work ethic. Generally speaking, traditionalists have a very strong work ethic and are willing to work hard for the goals of the company. They like to see a job done well; this means that the job has been completed and not done haphazardly. They like to take accountability for their work and want the outcome to reflect positively on them.

Boomers like work. In fact, they often live to work and are hard workers. They truly love to work hard and are personally gratified when they perform well at work. They are also very competitive in nature and like for their work to be done the best and before anyone else's is finished. The pride they take in their work is often evident in the outcome of what they are working on. This generation also likes to have a strong performance and not something just slapped together.

Xers work because it is usually a necessity; remember that they are always looking for work-life balance and for the personal benefit of the work that they are doing. Xers do like to work hard, but in return they usually want something for themselves, such as job security, good pay, promotions, flexible schedules, and so on. However, for Xers this comes at a price, because they place strong emphasis on work-life balance. This group's members do like to turn in a good performance if it is something that they are passionate about. They do not like to be micromanaged through the process and instead want to produce something that has their mark on it. If the outcome is not done as well as it could have been, they are usually unfazed and willing to rework it to make it better.

Millennials can take work or leave it. Millennials get bored easily but are willing to work hard as long as they feel a benefit to them personally, such as career advancement or financial rewards. For this group's members, turning in a good performance means that all the variables must be in their favor: the right resources, the right team (remember, this group likes group processes and decisions), and the right reasons to do it. Be aware, however, that this generation sometimes has difficulty taking accountability for their actions and work, so a poor performance might not be "their fault."

Because each generation uses its own value system as the bar from which to measure the others, the differences in the quality of performance or work ethic (or the lack thereof) can cause conflict and tension among the generations. As the nurse manager, you must be clear about the expectations so that everyone knows the goal. Do not accept anything less than what you qualified as the minimum level of performance; certainly, do not settle for poor-quality work.

To maximize the quality of care on each shift, it is essential that charge nurses know the strengths and weaknesses of every nurse on their shift and make assignments accordingly. To help ensure that every patient always receives the best care possible, it is also a good practice to sign resource/lunch buddies based on complementary strengths. Creating an environment where your staff is engaged is half the battle. A culture of self-awareness and generational harmony is the best foundation that you can build for your department; from that, they can go forward and do their thing.

WHICH GENERATION IS THE MOST PRODUCTIVE?

Traditionalists 17%, boomers 45%, Xers 32%, and millennials 6%, according to a Harris Interactive survey of 3,868 adults ages 21 to 83 (Charles Schwab & Age Wave, 2008).

Coaching

Coaching is a good strategy to increase performance and teach new skills. Of course, like everything that we have talked about in this book, nurse managers must account for generational differences when coaching staff. Clearly, some strategies are more effective when coaching specific generations (Table 4.2).

TABLE 4.2
COACHING TIPS

MOTIVATING THE VARIOUS GENERATIONS	
Traditionalists	Be tactful.
	Respect privacy.
	Build rapport.
	Be respectful.
	Ask permission to coach.
	They consider no news is good news.
Boomers	Be tactful.
	Create harmony and agreement.
	Use questions rather than statements.
	Treat as equals.
	Provide yearly feedback with documentation.
Xers	Be direct and honest.
	They value equity and fairness.
	Be relaxed and informal.
	Provide regular feedback, focused on their performance.
Millennials	They like public recognition.
	Develop trust.
	Be direct and honest.
	Show confidence.
	Treat them like an adult.
	They need structure.
	They crave continuous feedback.

(ICHRN, 2009)

When it comes to coaching Xers and millennials, it is important to be consistent and to respect them as individuals. The benefits and rewards need to be known upfront so that they can determine whether the objective is worth it. You should also provide large amounts of flexibility and freedom of time and opinions. Skill development is very important to these groups. They will sometimes take a job with lower pay to learn another skill set (if they think it will meet their needs later). Working through change isn't a problem with these groups, but it has affected their loyalty. Empowerment is a strong tool, too, because it is important to Xers and millennials, who value the opportunity to participate in shared governance, self-scheduling, and job sharing (Marshburn & Scott, 2009).

Baby boomers and millennials complement each other well in coaching situations. This is primarily because the age gap lends itself to a parent/child type of situation, which is gratifying to both cohorts (Kennedy, 1996). When coaching millennials, it is important to balance both the give and take, meaning what you ask them to do and what you are willing to do for them. Both managers and coaches should work hard to make them feel important, just like their parents and family did while they were growing up. If you don't acquiesce and do this, it will make things more difficult later.

To meet the coaching needs of millennials, provide more feedback than you are used to; remember, this is a group where everyone got trophies, so they are used to and need regular feedback. We catered to this generation to prevent hard feelings and make them all feel good about themselves, but that set them up to be ill prepared for the work world. Not everyone gets promoted or advances as they hoped in their career, which means that someone wins and someone loses (or as we now say, *doesn't win*). Sometimes there is difficult news to deliver in the workplace. Astute nurse managers know this in advance and can choose their words carefully when delivering bad news, and maybe even come up with an attractive consolation prize (such as training, development, or coaching).

Help coach millennials to think independently, because this is a generation that likes group think and group decision making. You should also be mindful that this group is getting parental career advice on a continual basis (Alsop, 2011). Respect the advice the millennials are receiving from family and friends; after all, you don't want to be the topic of conversation at Sunday dinner.

Xers like to be coached with more of a hands-off approach, so suggest what needs to be accomplished and let them work through how to do it. Although this is clearly more of a distant technique, they still consider this coaching. They are very industrious and will respond well to this approach. Don't worry, either; they will ask for help if they need it. However, boomers like to be coached by being provided with the expectations and even some suggestions on how to accomplish the goal. They will then try out the options and work through the objectives in a way that allows them to both break some rules and follow others to meet their comfort level. Although traditionalists prefer to be told what to do, they are hard, methodical workers who will get it done.

Coaching of boomers and traditionalists is often best done by their same generation or by these two generations coaching each other. Both share a sense of commitment to the workplace and to the team; they also share a similar work ethic. These two generations appreciate honest feedback delivered in a constructive and resourceful manner.

Mentoring

Mentoring is another great way to help different nurses of any generation transition to changes in their environment, whether it is onboarding a new nurse or mentoring a new charge nurse. Mentoring is also a strong way to develop staff personally and professionally. As Billy Brown, Past President of Sigma Theta Tau said, "The opportunity to mentor another nurse is an honor, privilege and is a personally rewarding" (Brown, n.d.; Cary, 2008.).

Intergenerational mentoring works well when the two parties are well matched. So, combining a traditionalist or a boomer with a millennial is a good fit, but matching a traditionalist with an Xer is not such a good fit. These pairings work, because traditionalists like to share their expertise and history. Millennials see this as grandparent-like, and because they have strong family relationships, this is a natural fit. However, Xers see this as more cumbersome and meddling and not as helpful. In addition, boomers are more like the millennials' parents, so although millennials are comfortable in that relationship, this may not necessarily a good fit, because the millennials are trying to learn their own way of doing things. Mentoring Xers is difficult, but not impossible; it's all about the personalities.

> **NOTE**
>
> *Mentoring should share, educate, and inspire so that the mentoring relationship benefits both parties.*

To have enough well-prepared nurse leaders in the future, mentoring is very important for succession planning. Intergenerational mentoring is an effective way to develop the mentors as well as the mentorees. Mentorship of future leaders can help share accountability of succession planning and foster an environment of respectful dialogue, honesty, and integrity as it pertains to sharing opinions and articulating differences (Cary, 2008).

Millennials are used to frequent parental guidance and view mentoring as helpful. This group's members also tend to feel entitled to special treatment and believe that they need direct access to senior leaders and organization executives. Mentoring provides structure for these interactions.

Training and Development

Staff training and development are important components of sharing up-to-date knowledge and retaining your employees. Millennials place a high value on education and development. According to the American Society for Training & Development, more than 41% of inadequately trained employees leave their employers within their first year, whereas only 12% of employees with excellent training and development opportunities leave within their first year. Of course, *inadequate* and *adequate* are defined by the survey participants, and millennials have a critical eye when it comes to training. Investing in millennials is smart; by doing so, you increase the odds of keeping them, and their additional knowledge will likely eventually contribute to the organization. As Cam Marston, a well-known generational expert, puts it, "Training enhances profits, improves the organization's competitive edge, increases worker productivity and increases employee satisfaction and retention" (Marston, 2012).

The question shouldn't be whether to train. Instead, it should just be a "question of deciding the topics" (Marston, 2012). Remember, this group's members are looking for broad skill sets that they can take with them *when* they move on, essentially skill portability. Don't make them wait until they have paid their dues; they are impatient and will become disengaged and just leave. Start training upon orientation and continue it throughout their tenure with your organization (Marston, 2012).

Because each of the generations learns differently, it is essential that you know how to effectively train each generational group—not just adult learning principles, but how to truly engage and get through to your audience so that it sinks in. Each generation has educational tools that seem to work better for it as well as specific learning preferences (Table 4.3). Therefore, you might have to customize your training. You may even have to adapt your style or format several times for the same content. Just ensure that the message resonates with the audience.

TABLE 4.3
LEARNING DIFFERENCES

	Learn Best Through	Learning Tools	Learning Preferences (Likes)	Key Takeaway
Tradition- alists	Classroom lectures and presentations. Person-to-person interaction. Hands-on and role playing.	Important to read and understand policies.	Like to share their expertise.	Avoid situations where they may lose face.
Boomers	Structured learning environment and programs that address individual learning needs.	Enjoy problem-solving activities. Like to know steps of the process.	Like to role play and talk through scenarios.	Allow safe environment for questions or disagreements. Handle with respect.

Xers	Multimedia; break up presentations with graphics, interaction, and video clips.	Fast-paced classroom environments and simulated experiences are good. Want to figure things out on their own.	Like individual learning exercises and self-paced computer/ online learning.	Provide many stimuli during class; you can even provide more than one at a time.
Millennials	Supervised, structured environment. Like internships, capstone experiences, and coaching/ mentoring (provides comfort and safety net).	Independent, fast-paced learning environments, including simulation and learning games.	Like self-paced computer/ online learning. Enjoy group learning exercises.	They like to hit the ground running and don't want to put in as much time to move up. Learning from seasoned nurses is seen as a faster track to the top.

(Halfer, 2007)

Learning styles and preferences vary among the generations. Here are some helpful tips for delivering training content:

- Millennials tend to prefer short snippets, such as Internet video clips, for their educational content. You may have to string many snippets together to deliver all the required content. Be aware of the need to mix modalities; incorporate video clips with classroom projects and hands-on sessions. Millennials simply cannot "do" a 60- to 90-minute didactic lecture. They cannot sit still or stay off their phones that long. So, break it up by offering video clips, web-based games, computer-based learning modules, or personal stories from real frontline workers. No matter what you do, keep it interesting so that they don't disengage (Marston, 2012).

- Xers like to be in control, so DVDs or video clips work well; they can fast-forward through what they think they don't need. Mixed modalities are also good with this group. Just remember that they don't like to feel lectured to. They also like frequent breaks to check phones and e-mails; otherwise, they will just check them during the training.

- Baby boomers prefer classroom settings where they can ask questions and receive personal attention. In-person settings with dialogue and hands-on activities are best for this group. They like role playing, repetition, and getting the hang of it before they transition back to the department.

- Traditionalists like the classroom setting to engage in discussion about a given topic so that they can talk about it and make sure they understand it. Role playing also works well with this group; they want to be comfortable with the new skill set before leaving training.

Creative nurse managers may even develop a departmental website and post educational links here for future self-exploration, which will appeal to the Xers and millennials.

Succession Planning

Approximately 20% of the current nursing leaders are eligible for retirement. By 2020, this number will grow to nearly 75% (Westbrook, 2012). Many leadership vacancies will likely not have any up-and-coming leaders standing in line to fill the position. Many baby boomers are in current leadership roles, and when they go, so does much of our organizational knowledge base. This will have a significant impact on nursing and health care as a whole.

Xers are bringing up the rear on leadership, but they do not have as quite as much experience as the baby boomers, and they often entered nursing later in life; catching up might prove difficult. However, older Xers are very strong managers and will be suitable alternatives to keep our well-oiled machines functioning. A looming concern, though, is that many Xers and millennials have no experience of the stress of being on call 24/7, working long hours, dealing with the day-to-day crises, juggling competing priorities, and dealing with lack of support. So, regardless of any financial rewards, many will be unwilling to move into leadership roles. In fact, the leadership pool might be small, while the advance practice nurse pool continues to grow ever larger. Ask millennial nurses what they want to do, and they will tell you that they plan to be an advance practice nurse of some sort. What have we done?

Succession planning means having identified specific staff in mind for key positions as they become vacant. Ideally, these staff should be receiving mentoring and coaching along the way, improving their chances of success with increased responsibilities in the future. As nurse managers, we need to seek out early on individuals who exhibit a desire to lead so that we can begin the coaching process as soon as possible. As a profession rooted in tradition, we need to get over the old-school notion that nurses must put in their time. In fact, most millennials believe that putting in their time should take no more than 3 years. Xers and millennials aren't patient enough to wait longer than that; they'll lose interest and move on in the meantime. This may mean moving to another unit/department, moving to a different hospital, or perhaps even getting out of patient care altogether. Younger nurses know that nursing is a highly sought-after skill set in many other fields.

NOTE

Our profession and our patients cannot afford for a migration of nurses to other careers. As nurse managers, the challenge is how to get the training, development, and experience to these groups in less than 3 years.

Succession planning should be viewed from each nurse leader's vantage point. This means that chief nursing officers should have plans for all of their direct reports as well as for hard-to-fill or key nursing positions. Nurse managers should have succession plans for their direct reports, unit/department-based leaders, and shift supervisors/charge nurses. Developing a succession plan for each director, manager, and supervisor is essential to the smooth, long-term operation of any health care organization. Make sure that your organization provides opportunities for formal/informal leadership and ensure that trained mentors, preceptors, and coaches are standing ready to make the experience as positive and successful as possible. Here is a simple four-step process:

The first step is to get a sense of which positions will need to be replaced and in what time frame. You can use a simple spreadsheet tool to document the annual risk assessment as part of a leadership exercise to provide insight to future needs. A good time for a personal conversation with current nurse leaders is during their annual evaluation. The discussion of future personal and professional goals is important for growth and development purposes. Nurse leaders have a sense of their plans, just maybe not all the details. They might not be willing to share many details, but learn what you can; it will help you make a plan. This conversation should be held by nurse managers with their supervisors, charge nurses, and current nursing staff. As a picture begins to emerge about the upcoming leadership needs, an organizational nurse leader succession plan can be developed.

The topics to prompt discussion should include some of the following:

- Where do you see yourself in 1, 3, 5, 10 years?

- What do you want to do with this experience?

- What is your ideal role?

- Are you interested in advancing your education?

- Do you want to move up in the organization, system, network, corporation? (for higher-level positions)

- Are you able to relocate? (for higher-level positions)

After the risk assessment has been completed and the status of all nurse leaders is known, a succession plan can be developed for each position of concern, which should be rolled up into a larger organizational nurse leader succession plan.

The second step is that for each position included in the plan, the identification of the skills necessary to be successful in the role should be outlined. The nurse manager learning domain framework (AONE, 2006) indicates that key competencies include financial management, human resource management, performance improvement, foundation thinking skills, strategic management, clinical practice knowledge, accountability, career planning, relationship management, and influencing others. You might require very specific and unique skills necessary for each nurse manager, charge nurse, and supervisor to succeed in that particular role in your organization.

The third step should include and assessment of internal talent. When evaluating your current nursing staff, are there middle or high performers with potential who desire development and advancement? Do you have staff who are likely to stay with the organization and who are champions and role models and would make good successors?

The fourth step should include the actual development of the future leaders. You can do this done through a variety of means, either internal training or external training, depending on the resources of your organization. Organizations that invest in broad-based leadership training can usually identify potential leaders, because they tend to rise to the top through their performance in their units/departments, committee work, or projects.

Action plans can be used to organize development activities, follow time lines, and track progress. For action plans to be effective, the nurse manager should engage the participant in the development. Any discussion and negotiation should occur at this stage. The goals should be clearly identified and aligned with the overall purpose of the plan. There should also be discussion and progress reports regularly, twice each year at a minimum. There should also be rewards or benefits for participating, such as the occasional opportunity to function as a charge nurse, admit nurse, and so on, to diversify the learning process. Keeping future leaders engaged and learning is paramount to creating adequate leadership bench strength.

WHAT MAKES YOUR GENERATION UNIQUE?
Boomers
Work ethic 17%
Respectful 14%
Values 8%
Baby boomers 6%
Smarter 5%

© 2010 Pew Research Center

Career Advancement

Setting staff up to advance their careers is not only rewarding for them but can also be very gratifying for the manager. Observational or shadowing experiences are often helpful for nurses to either rule in or rule out a potential career path. At any point in their careers, nurses may determine that they are interested in leadership. As a nurse manager, observational or shadowing experiences provide a good way to introduce nurses to the real world of leadership. These are much less intense than an internship and often give you, as well as the observer, a test drive of what this position *really* does in the course of a day or week; they give you a pretty good idea about the level of interest of the observer as well. You may even learn the answer as to whether you should invest in succession planning for this person.

The step up from an observation or shadowing experience is an internship. Internships provide a good sense of what a job truly entails. Internships provide hands-on, experience-based learning. These typically occur through a structured academic program and should have goals and objectives established before the start of the experience. It is also common practice to assign the intern a project and to expect a high-quality deliverable at the culmination of the internship experience.

For nurse managers, succession planning needs to be a priority and an annual event. It cannot be done one time for an upcoming crisis. It should not be a popularity contest and should not be based on playing favorites. Instead, it should provide objective and well-thought-out plans, matching strengths and needs (Kowske, 2009). Understanding the differences among the generations will help you determine your strong successors for a variety of nursing leadership positions, including charge nurse, supervisor, manager, director, or even chief nursing officer.

Organizations will have to replace the typical career ladder we are used to with a career matrix or lattice for Xers and millennials. This new approach allows for movement upward and from side to side and even allows for career pauses as needed when significant life events, such as marriage or having a baby, occur. Xers and millennials are motivated to advance their careers and work hard as long as there is something in it for them and it fits with their need for work-life balance, whereas traditionalists and boomers are motivated by desire to improve performance. The tips listed in Table 4.4 help mitigate generational nuances when motivating employees provide nurse managers with a road map for success. Xers and millennials are more of a challenge to motivate and are looking for motivators that provide them what they are searching for: opportunity, flexibility, and respect (Table 4.5).

TABLE 4.4
MOTIVATING THE VARIOUS GENERATIONS

Traditionalists	Use a personal touch (handwritten notes, calls).
	Provide traditional perks.
	Use them as mentors.
	Reward is a job well done.
Boomers	Personal relationships are important.
	Offer public recognition.
	Provide work perks.
	Give name recognition (quote them in newsletters).
	Reward hours worked and effort.
	Talk about legacy.
	Like involvement/participation.
	Public recognition is their reward.
Xers	Provide opportunities to develop skills.
	Provide opportunities for promotion.
	Give them multiple tasks and projects.
	Give feedback, but do not micromanage.
	Allow some laxness.
	Freedom is a reward.

Millennials	Provide competitive pay and benefits.
	Ensure a good environment.
	Show opportunities for advancement.
	Provide career planning and counseling.
	Offer ways to be socially conscious.
	Reward is meaningful work.

(ICHRN, 2009)

TABLE 4.5
ADDITIONAL TIPS FOR MOTIVATING XERS AND MILLENNIALS

Xers	Ensure that schedules promote work-life balance.
	Employ hands-off supervision. (Tell me what to do, and I will get it done.)
	Are practical. Allow them to figure things out for themselves.
	Do not provide too much structure. (They often find organizational more irritating.)
	Want development, but in bullet points and bite-size pieces.
	Allow them to balance their own needs and roam in their careers.
Millennials	Love team work, so allow them to work together on projects.
	Well educated, so include them in the big picture.
	Have a can-do attitude and like complex issues to resolve.

(Marshburn & Scott, 2009; Marston, 2012)

TIME-SAVING TOOL

Hallway conversations and "rounding" on your staff throughout the year will help you identify staff interests and goals. You can keep this information in mind as positions or need arises in your facility.

Summary

Generation-specific interventions for the various phases of career advancement, from transition, performance, and up to succession planning, is a skill set that nurse managers should learn and embrace. Because the nurse manager does the initial selection of staff, it makes sense that the nurse manager is also directly involved with the development and success of each individual staff member. Over time, this will become more natural and comfortable for the nurse manager and should evolve into a mutually beneficial exercise for both the staff member and the department.

Differences between the generations in socialization, coaching, training, and orientation can lead to misunderstandings, conflict, and mistrust. Therefore, understanding the value systems and goals of each generation, encouraging teamwork and building a culture where retention can thrive, needs a dedicated and creative nurse manager. With this knowledge, you can enhance your skills to deliver what you and your staff need to be successful.

References

Alsop, R. (2011). How the millennial generation is shaking up the workplace. *Workforce Management/The Right Thing.*

American Hospital Association (AHA). (2010). Workforce 2015: Strategy trumps shortage. Retrieved from http://www.aha.org/content/00-10/workforce2015report.pdf

American Organization of Nurse Executives (AONE). (2006). AONE supports the Insititute of Medicine's recommendations on the future of nursing. Retrieved from http://nurseleader.com

Brown, B. (n.d.). Board leadership development program. Retrieved from http://www.nursingsociety.org/ LeadershipInstitute/omada/pages/omada_main.aspx

Cary, S. (2008). Mentoring generations today for tomorrow's leaders. *Nephrology Nursing Journal, 35*(2), 118–119.

Charles Schwab & Age Wave. (2008). Rethinking retirement: Four american generations share their views on life's third act. Retrieved from http://www.agewave.com/research/ SchwabAgeWaveRethinkingRetirement071508.pdf

Cowin, L. S., & Hengstberger-Sims, C. (2006). New graduate nurse self-concept and retention: A longitudinal survey. *International Journal of Nursing Studies, 43*(1), 59–70.

Dunton, N., Gajewski, B., Klaus, S., & Pierson, B. (2007). The relationship of nursing workforce characteristics to patient outcomes. *Online Journal of Issues in Nursing, 12*(3). Retrieved from http://www.nursingworld.org/ MainMenuCategories/ANAMarketplace/ANAPeriodicals/ OJIN/TableofContents/Volume122007/No3Sept07/ NursingWorkforceCharacteristics.aspx

Halfer, D. (2007). A magnetic strategy for new graduate nurses. *Nursing Economic$, 25*(1), 6–12.

Henderson, A., Fox, R., & Malko-Nyhan, K. (2006). An evaluation of preceptors' perceptions of educational preparation and organizational support for their role. *Journal of Continuing Education in Nursing, 37*(3), 130–136.

International Centre for Human Resources in Nursing (ICHRN). (2009). Managing the multi-generational nursing workforce. *Managerial and Policy Implications*, white paper.

The Joint Commission. (2004). *Sentinel events: Cause and planning improvement, 2nd edition.* Chicago, IL: The Joint Commission.

Keller, J. L., Meekins, K., & Summers, B. L. (2006). Pearls and pitfalls of a new graduate academic residency program. *Journal of Nursing Administration, 36*(12), 589–598.

Kennedy, M. (1996). Boomers and busters: Ways to bridge the gap. *Kennedy's Career Strategist.*

Kenward, K., & Zhong, E. (2006). *Report of findings from the Practice and Professional Issues survey: Fall 2004*. Chicago, IL: National Council of State Boards of Nursing.

Kowske, B. R. (2009). Millennials' (lack of) attitude problem: An empirical examination of generational effects on work attitudes. White paper, 1–15.

Lee, T., Tzeng, W., Lin, C., & Yeh, M. (2009). Effects of a preceptorship programme on turnover rate, cost, quality and professional development. *Journal of Clinical Nursing, 18*(8), 1217-1225.

Marshburn, D. M., & Scott, E. S. (2009). New nurses are not all alike: Meeting diverse transition needs of newly licensed nurses. Presentation.

Marston, C. (2012). *How to train millennials*. Mobile: Generational Insights.

Morrow, S. (2009). New graduate transitions: Leaving the nest, joining the flight. *Journal of Nursing Management, 17*, 278–287.

Pew Research Center. (2010). *Pew Social & Demographic Trends*. Pew Charitable Trust. Retrieved from http:\\pewresearch.org\pubs\1501\millennials-new-survey-generational-personality-upbeat-open-new-ideas-technology-bound

Satran, P. (2009). *How not to act old*. New York: HarperCollins Publishers.

Scott, E. S, Keehner Engelke, M., & Swanson, M. (2008). New nurse transitioning: Necessary or nice? *Applied Nursing Research, 21*(2), 75–83.

Thompson, J. W. (2004). J. Walter Thompson Specialized Communications for University of Michigan Health System. Lenexa, KS.

Westbrook, G. (2012, February). Succession planning in nursing who are tomorrow's leaders? *Nurse.com*, 42–47.

Wisotzkey, S. (2011). Will they stay or will they go? Insight into nursing turnover. *Nursing Management, 42*(2), 15–17.

5

Recruitment and Retention Strategies

Each generation imagines itself to be more intelligent than the one that went before it, and wiser than the one that comes after it.

–George Orwell

The four generations have all had different experiences with the recruitment process throughout the years. Searching for jobs today is totally different from what it was 5 or 10 years ago, let alone 80 years ago, when many traditionalists were seeking employment. Today, when we recruit, we use technology and post positions online on recruitment and job aggregation sites (for example, Monster.com) or social media sites. Years ago, jobs were listed in the newspaper classified ads, and prior to that we posted Help Wanted signs in windows. As nurse managers, you need to know how to work with your recruiters to reach the market that you are targeting.

Retention has also come to the forefront of a nurse manager's responsibilities. Retention used to just mean that you were staying with your employer as you had planned. But younger generations have come to realize that they have more choices and options, which means that employers have to actually work hard to keep their employees. Your role as a nurse manager is to create a work environment that engages all of your staff and results in a high-retention culture. This requires you to be innovative and flexible so that you can adapt to changing workforce needs and employee demands. Although much variation exists among the generations with regard to recruiting, hiring, and retaining employees, there are still some similarities, as well.

This chapter covers:

- How to recruit the various generations
- Helicopter parents
- Generation-specific retention tactics

Recruitment

The employment market has changed significantly over the years, affecting the various generations differently. Because of job scarcity and either living through or remembering the Great Depression, traditionalists worked very hard just to find a job. When they did find one, they usually held it for a long period of time. Boomers found a competitive market that needed more skilled workers and worked hard to advance their careers. Xers entered the workforce during a period of unusually low unemployment rates and became accustomed to a job market where the applicant is in a favorable position relative to the organization. As a result, Xers tend to believe that they can be selective when choosing employers/jobs and should be offered additional incentives by employers to work for them. Millennial employees are driven to seek new challenges and apply for positions that interest them, knowing that they can change a position if it isn't to their liking. Early millennials had a strong job market to choose from, but in the past 3 to 5 years, the job market has dried up, and job options have become fewer. Today, many college-educated millennials are underemployed but happy just to be working.

> **NOTE**
>
> *Organizations are now entering an entirely new recruitment world, with much of that change attributable to generational differences in the workforce.*

As a nurse manager, you need to treat your employees as your most valuable resource, while realizing that the acquisition and management of quality employees will be the most expensive and important issue you will face (Klinvex, 2012). You also need to anticipate future retirements in your department and plan to offset those by making sure that your department is attractive to younger nurses. As a nurse manager, your role is to identify the best nurses for your department, not only through interviews but also through the informal network of word of mouth among your existing employees. If you have to entice employees from another area, it is much more acceptable to poach staff from other facilities rather than from other departments. Identifying and acquiring the *right* staff to meet your goals is a long-term process and requires careful thought and planning.

Younger workers have different priorities and expectations compared to those who are leaving the workforce. Therefore, the tactics used to recruit millennials should play specifically to their expectations and interests. You need to carefully consider each vacant position and what market you want to pursue with your recruitment efforts. For example, if you are recruiting for a highly technical, procedural-based position such as Cardiac Cath Lab or Electrophysiology, you likely want to go after techies (a bit of a generalization, but most likely true). To find them, you need to post where they look, such as cardiology or cardiovascular sites, interventional blogs, and even medical device blogs/websites or social media sites.

Recruitment is a hands-on function that requires nurse managers to be personally involved, even if you have a recruitment department that provides this function. Ask your recruiters how they are going to recruit. What media are they using? Will there be a Facebook site? Can your department produce its own YouTube clip? Realize that the secret weapon here is that your current employees are the best recruiters that you have. Treat your employees well, keep them up-to-date on departmental happenings, and involve them in the pursuit of your department's goals; you will then have great word-of-mouth recruiters. Remember, they want good people to work with them, so they are invested in this, too. But in general, there are some helpful recruitment strategies, as identified below.

Recruitment Strategies
Traditionalists

As employees, traditionalists are hard workers, have strong skill sets, and are highly valued in the workplace. Because of the physical nature of nursing, such as lifting and transferring patients and patients' expectations of speed, the job often becomes more difficult for nurses as they age. However, we need to hire and retain this generation as long as we can. If you have positions that you think might be well suited for these employees, such as part-time positions or nursing roles that are less physical in nature, internal job-posting boards, word of mouth, and the classified ads are still the way to go for this bunch. Make sure that your job postings include messages that speak to traditional work values.

Boomers

This cohort has become much more comfortable with technology over time and typically now uses the Internet for job searches. Any job postings should speak directly to them and recognize their career accomplishments with some type of reward (for example, higher salary commensurate with experience, longevity bonuses, or supervisor roles). This group still likes to network and attend job fairs. They are excited by opportunities to mentor, coach, and share their experiences and expertise.

Xers

This group uses the Internet to search for positions and craves information, so its members are fairly sophisticated in terms of how and where they search. If they see a vacancy on a job aggregator site, they might also go to the organization-specific website. Then they'll likely move on to Facebook and YouTube to check out all aspects of the positions and the organization. Make sure to give this group's members a realistic preview of the job so that they know what to expect before they accept it. It is also good to let the team members spend some time with the applicants and even provide a tour of the department so that prospective employees can ask questions directly of their potential team members. Because of the importance of the work-life balance for this group, self-scheduling is a big draw for Xers.

Millennials

Millennials comprise more than 20% of today's population, and they are starting to prove their value in the workforce. The challenge for you is how to attract these eager and innovative individuals. The top five things that millennials look for in a job are as follows (Douglas, 2012):

- Work-life balance
- Having their voices heard
- Regular recognition
- A fun environment
- A collaborative team

Meaningful work is also important to this group. This group always has its eyes and ears open for "better" opportunities, such as more flexible schedules, more money, or just something that sparks an interest above and beyond what it is currently doing. Remember, they need to be challenged and to feel like they are doing something meaningful; otherwise, they will change jobs pretty quickly. This group searches for jobs on job aggregator sites and also searches on social media sites, such as Facebook and YouTube. This generational cohort is also very likely to check out its potential employers on a variety of sites to validate it is are reading/hearing. Word of mouth proves very effective with this group as well, especially referral bonus programs. Refer to Table 5.1 for more recruitment tips.

TABLE 5.1
GENERATION-SPECIFIC RECRUITMENT TIPS

Traditionalists	Don't rule them out yet.
	Look at them for part-time positions.
	Stress their valuable experience.
	Be very courteous and respectful.
	Use messages that speak to traditional values and work.

Boomers	Acknowledge their vast experience.
	Establish a challenge.
	Stress humane and positive working environment.
	Give them credit and respect for their previous achievements.
	Show them how to be a star in your organization
Xers	Emphasize balance.
	Discuss expected organizational changes.
	Create a fun, intimate work environment.
	Emphasize technology.
	Emphasize independence and flexibility in scheduling.
Millennials	Sell the organization.
	Show the opportunities for growth.
	Emphasize the organization's importance .
	Sell them on the job.
	Sell them on the organization's standing in the community and appeal to their sense of civic responsibility.
	Customize job opportunities.
	Emphasize flexibly.

Helicopter Parents

A relatively new phenomenon, known as *helicopter parents*, has generated a lot of attention lately. This term refers to parents who are overinvolved in their children's lives (even their professional lives). Helicopter parents *hover* (hence the term) incessantly, showing up to job interviews, insisting they be involved in negotiating salaries and benefits, and even demanding to sit in on annual evaluations or disciplinary actions. This is an extension of the role that these protective parents have played during the course of their millennial children's lives. They are doing what they do best, influencing outcomes for the benefit of their children. (Some large financial and accounting firms even provide parents of millennial employees with their own memory sticks of company benefits to review and host "bring your parents to work" days.)

As a nurse manager, the best way to handle helicopter parents is to set clear ground rules. If parents become too involved in their children's interactions with you, make sure to notify your human resources department. In addition, make it abundantly clear that the employee is who you will be dealing with and that any communication to the parents must come from their children. However, so as to not offend either your employees or their parents, you need to deliver this message in a sensitive, respectful manner.

> **NOTE**
>
> *Be careful, however, not to alienate either your millennial employees or their parents. An offended parent could translate into an upset employee who soon leaves to find a more sensitive organization.*

Retention

Why is retention so important? Two reasons really: Turnover is expensive, and it can be unsafe. The economic impact of nurse turnover is staggering, at a cost of $62,000 to $145,000 per nurse, depending on his or her specialty area. Note, as well, that every 1% increase in the turnover rate represents an additional organizational cost of $300,000 annually (Jones & Gates, 2007; Jones, 2008; Bowles & Candela, 2005), thus making sustained nurse turnover costs prohibitive to health care organizations. The constant churning compounds an already complex cost-containment environment for most health care organizations. Chapter 4, "Transition, Performance Management, and Succession Planning," discussed the patient-safety implications of high turnover, such as a higher number of falls and pressure ulcers.

We know that nurses leave their jobs for a variety of reasons. We see older nurses retire or decrease their hours; younger nurses become bored or disenchanted and move on. All in all, retention is still problematic among younger nurses: First-year turnover is 30%, and second-year nurse turnover is even worse at 57% to 66% (Aiken, Clarke, Sloane, Sochalski, Busse, Clarke, & Shamian, 2001; Bowles & Candela, 2005; Wieck, Dols, & Landrum, 2010; Wisotzkey, 2011). In addition, two-thirds of nurses under age 30 plan to leave their jobs within 5 years (Bowles & Candela, 2005; Wieck, Dols, & Landrum, 2010). To validate this, another study of 1,773 nurses found that 33% of millennial nurses plan to leave their positions within the next 2 years. This increased to 66% of millennial nurses who plan to leave within 5 years, even though they indicated that they are highly satisfied with their jobs. These numbers demonstrate why the transition of new nurses is so important to the early establishment of commitment to the organization.

One has to ask whether turnover is higher among millennial nurses compared to millennials employed in other industries. Yes. By comparison, overall first-year millennial turnover for all industries is only 16%, compared to 30% to 33% in nursing. In addition, only 24% of all millennials leave their jobs after 2 years, compared to 55% to 57% of new nurses (Marston, 2010, 2012; Bowles & Candela, 2005; Wisotzkey, 2011).

As nurse managers, we should be very concerned that so many nurses plan to leave their current positions even though they are highly satisfied with their jobs. This fact indicates that we still have opportunities to work on retention in nursing. Retaining our younger nurses is essential not only to improve our current turnover rates but also to continue to build the pipeline of youth in nursing so that there is a cadre of younger nurses to grow and develop to advance the profession as a whole. We need to get serious about fixing retention now; after all, in just a few years, millennials will make up the majority of the workforce, and then it will be even more difficult.

Retention Strategies

Dealing with the retention of multiple generations requires creativity, because what is important to one group might not be remotely important to another. Each group has its own needs, values, and concerns. Therefore, retention strategies must be specific to the individual. I have provided some retention strategies for you broken down by generation.

Traditionalists

One study demonstrated that traditionalists are looking for flexibility, fitness, stress, pay, and morale, meaning that the presence of these factors will likely increase the odds of traditionalists remaining in their positions for a few more years (ICHRN, 2009):

- *Flexibility* refers to their position being a part-time or shared position to better meet their employment needs. They also have a strong preference for flextime and school-year-term employment, such as 9 months on and 3 months off, to travel or care for grandkids.

- *Fitness* refers to working in areas of reduced stress/ workload or even working in roles that include less lifting and physical activity.

- *Stress* refers to the perceived staffing shortages and amount of work compared to the amount of time to complete it.

- *Pay* needs to be commensurate with their experience and, in their opinion, fair.

- *Morale* means that this group is valued by its peers for its contributions at work.

WHAT MAKES YOUR GENERATION UNIQUE?

Traditionalists
  WWII, Great Depression 14%
  Smarter 13%
  Honest 12%
  Work ethic 10%

© 2010 Pew Research Center

Boomers

Although much focus has been placed on retaining millennial nurses and improving the workplace for traditionalists, it is the midcareer nurses, boomers, and Xers whom we should be working hard to keep. These are typically our nurses with 5 to 20 years of experience; they are very knowledgeable and often among our highest performers. A 2011 study of nearly 100 mid-career nurses with more than 10 years of experience found that the *most* important factors for them to remain with their current employers were positive work environment, pay, benefits, continuing education, and flexible scheduling. The *least* important factors to mid-career nurses are career-advancement opportunities, full-time work opportunities, and opportunities for specialization (McGillis Hall, LaLonde, Dales, Peterson, & Cripps, 2011). The lessons here are that access to good mentors, accommodations, life balance, helpful colleagues, and continuing-education opportunities are desirable and will promote retention among this group. Develop retention plans for this generational group with this in mind.

Xers

Xers have been ominously looking forward to, in a vulture-like way, the retirement of boomers so that they can begin to assume the roles that boomers have held for so long. However, as retirements continue to be put off by boomers, Xers continue to grow increasingly more impatient with their opportunities, as they sense the window of opportunity closing ever so slowly. As a nurse manager, placing Xers in succession-planning mode to afford them the opportunity for coaching and mentoring is viewed as a positive step in the right direction by this group and will keep its members around for a while longer. Involving them in succession planning and coaching opportunities will help slow their creep to the door. This group's members also make good mentors when matched well, and this too is a growth and development opportunity that will buy you some time. This group has a lot to offer and wants to be engaged in learning and mentoring opportunities. This generation also likes to be involved with decision making and sharing its opinion, so shared governance activities are helpful to retain this group as well. Remember that this group's member value independence, autonomy, and advancement in their careers, so focus your retention efforts around those key generational values.

Millennials

Because meaningful work is important to this group, you might think that nursing has an easier time with retention than some of the other professions. But don't take that for granted; you must continually remind this group of the good it is doing. Also remember that this generation is impatient and can't bear to think about putting its time in to earn a promotion. Generally, they see themselves moving up shortly after orientation and surely after no longer than 3 years. Growing up, this group became accustomed to 24/7 news channels and television, which has proved to them that things happen quickly in the world.

To millennials, even working for 2 years in one department seems like a lifetime (or a life sentence). Working for 5 or so years before being promoted to a manager or director is almost untenable. This creates an environment of high turnover. Unfairly, the turnover of millennials is misinterpreted as a lack of loyalty; it isn't intended to be that. Instead, they are just expressing their displeasure by voting with their feet. The attitude of millennials is often that if "I can't be at the top in 2 or 3 years, I am willing to go somewhere where I can move up faster," and they will make those career leaps that, in their opinion, will help them succeed faster. To avoid the constant churn that millennials can represent, managers need to think outside the traditional career-progression framework. This is a paradigm shift in nursing and will force nurse managers to do things very differently or risk losing your younger nurses.

One option that may show promise to retain these talented individuals is an accelerated program for leadership development. Although untraditional, it is not unreasonable to think that potential nurse leaders can be identified early on after the successful completion of orientation; then discussions can be held to determine their level of interest in such a program. Mentors are an important part of the success of this program, along with the appropriate education content in formats that optimize millennial learning. A 12-month program provides time for development and education to prepare for a transition into a charge nurse or supervisor role. This fast-track concept may appear troubling to traditionalists and boomers, as these young nurses didn't put their time in. However, millennials will welcome incremental increases in responsibility and progress. Investing in a fast track for charge-nurse/supervisor development might be more expensive than filling vacant charge-nurse roles in the typical manner, but losing the millennial nurse to turnover is altogether more expensive overall. Clearly, this is a generation gap; other generations see it as giving in to the younger and more-demanding nurses, and it contributes to the perception of the sense of entitlement that this cohort has. However, this may be a good way to retain your young and energetic nurses. Refer to Table 5.2 for generation-specific retention tactics.

TABLE 5.2
GENERATION-SPECIFIC RETENTION TACTICS

Traditionalists	Allow flexible schedules/shorter hours. Be creative; use 4- or 6-hour shifts.
	Provide devices to minimize physical demands (lifting devices, built-in bed scales, and so on).
	Facilitate gradual retirement from the patient-care arena when they are ready.
	Consider seasonal work to accommodate travel.
	Offer a personal touch; get to know them.
	Help others value and respect this group.
	Use experience to help mentor new staff.
	Establish organization-wide communication, with senior leaders attending department-specific meetings to talk with staff and learn firsthand the challenges facing managers and employees.
	Allow these nurses to move into roles as admission or discharge nurses, schedulers, or occupational/employee health nurses.
Boomers	Promote concept of slowly winding down versus retiring completely.
	Use experience to develop educational materials.
	Solicit them to step up and become supervisors, mentors, or preceptors.
	Consider seasonal work to accommodate travel (or even sabbaticals).

	Provide public recognition.
	Establish organization-wide communication, with senior leaders attending department-specific meetings to talk with staff and learn firsthand the challenges facing managers and employees.
Xers	Be aware that you have hard-working but short-term free agents on board.
	Provide frequent options and allow them to drive process.
	Consistently provide ample opportunities for training and learning new skills; allow job changes to not lose them.
	Provide flexibility to allow them to balance work and life.
	Communicate often and involve them in decisions (like shared governance).
	Do not micromanage (makes them want to shut down).
	Facilitate mediation, because Xers don't like conflict. (They will go a long time not speaking to someone.)
	Consider seasonal work and sabbaticals.
Millennials	Involve them in decisions.
	Provide lots of current/real-time feedback (does not have to be done in person).
	Incorporate lots of technology and chances to use real-time, web-based resources.
	Redesign jobs to be fun as well as rewarding.
	Build and develop their skill base. (They want portability.)
	Allow them to balance their workflow; they like to multitask and cross-train.
	Build flexibility and mobility into their career paths that also works for you; otherwise, they will leave to find it.
	Provide access to social networks.
	Allow time off to participate in their passion (social responsibility).
	Create an improved intranet site where employees and physicians can recognize one another for exceptional acts of caring, just one of many rewards and recognition activities.
	Schedule events and outings to build community.
	Establish organization-wide communication, with senior leaders attending department-specific meetings to talk with staff and learn firsthand the challenges facing managers and employees.

(Pettit, 2010)

Key Retention Motivators

To build and promote an overall culture of retention, you need to hard-wire the motivators that will retain employees in your department or organization. Five primary intrinsic human motivators provide a framework for creating this environment (Manion, 2005; ICHRN, 2009):

- Healthy interpersonal relationships
- Meaningful work
- A sense of competence or self-efficacy
- Having autonomy or choice
- The achievement of progress

Healthy Interpersonal Relationships

- This means healthy relationships among coworkers on all shifts, and even those in other departments with whom they interact.
- Define employees' responsibilities with regard to creating sustainable work relationships.
- Help your staff learn conflict resolution, feedback, and listening skills.

Meaningful Work

- Make sure that your employees understand the meaningful nature of their work.
- Share stories about how your staff positively impacts the lives of their patients/families.
- Engage your staff in ways to reduce redundant or nonvalue activities that they are engaged in regularly.

A Sense of Competence or Self-Efficacy

- Assign mentors to facilitate succession planning.
- Coach your staff to further develop their skills.
- Provide ongoing learning opportunities.

Having Autonomy or Choice

- Ask your staff for input and feedback and really listen to it.
- Utilize a departmental shared governance or participatory decision-making model.
- Allow for individual styles to influence their work, as long as standards are followed and the desired outcomes are attained.

The Achievement of Progress

- Recognize the small steps of progress as they occur.
- Monitor progress and demonstrate results.
- Celebrate accomplishments.

Summary

Recruitment for the different generations requires creativity and patience. Because of the dynamic workforce environment, you will continually be challenged to find the right way to reach your targeted audience. The biggest hurdle for a nurse manager is keeping ambitious employees from all generations motivated and engaged. Make sure to try the generation-specific tactics discussed in this chapter, and if something doesn't work, change it with something else. When it comes to fast-tracking millennials to leadership roles, we need to get past the notion of their leapfrogging others or being moved up undeservedly when the older generations had to put in more time for similar advancement. We need to get over it and welcome the potential of young nurses. After all, they might have what it takes to reach management sooner than we think.

This chapter covered the following:

- How to recruit the various generations

- Helicopter parents

- Generation-specific retention tactics

As a nurse manager, the responsibility of staffing your department with good people belongs to you. However, you don't have to reinvent the wheel; there are helpful tactics to improve recruitment and retention for areas under your control. Make sure to work closely with your recruiters, and don't be afraid to use innovative approaches to find the best staff for your department. Understand your targets, and try to recruit and retain and utilize generational-specific strategies and tactics. Retention is one of the most difficult metrics to improve on, because it requires frequent reinvention. However, it is important to keep a well-rounded group of staff nurses on your unit, as each makes his or her own special contributions. Traditionalists tend to be even keeled and have many years of experience under their belts, and boomers are often well-versed in politics and are good at keeping large groups relatively happy. This competitive bunch is also good at rallying the team to push for better quality scores as they don't like to lose, even light-hearted quality performance metric competitions. The Xers contribute innovation and motivation to continually try to become more efficient, and millennials are generally good at building relationships and making sure that everyone is included. Keeping your team together is tough work. Try the strategies and tactics outlined in this chapter to make positive strides in retention. It is not a one-time fix, though. Promoting a culture of retention requires ongoing time and attention. Don't give up. You can do it!

References

Aiken, L. H., Clarke, S. P., Sloane, D. M., Sochalski, J. A., Busse, R., Clarke, H., & Shamian, J. (2001). Nurses' reports on hospital care in five countries: The ways in which nurses' work is structured have left nurses among the least satisfied workers, and the problem is getting worse. *Health Affairs, 20*(3), 43–53.

Bowles, C., & Candela, L. (2005). First job experiences of recent RN graduates: Improving the work environment. *Nevada RNformation, 14*(2), 16–19.

Douglas, C. (2012). Motivating Gen Y. *Human Resource Management.* Accessed from www.hrmreport.com/article/ Motivating-Gen-Y/

International Centre for Human Resources in Nursing (ICHRN). (2009). Managing the multi-generational nursing workforce. *Managerial and Policy Implications*, white paper.

Jones, C. B. (2008). Revisiting nurse turnover costs: Adjusting for inflation. *Journal of Nursing Administration, 38*(1), 11–18.

Jones, C. B., & Gates, M. (2007). The costs and benefits of nurse turnover: A business case for nurse retention. *Online Journal of Issues in Nursing, 12*(3), Manuscript 4. Retrieved from http://ezproxy.uttyler.edu:2048/login?url=http://search. ebscohost.com.ezproxy.ttuhsc.edu/login.aspx?direct=true&d b=rzh&AN=2009867880&loginpage=Login.asp&site=ehost- live&scope=site

Klinvex, K. (2012). The next generation. *Human Resource Management.* Accessed from http://www.hrmreport.com/ article/The-Next-Generation/

Manion, J. (2005). *Create a positive health care workplace: Practical strategies to retain today's workforce and find tomorrow's.* Chicago, IL: AHA Press.

Marston, C. (2010). *Generational insights: Practical solutions for understanding and engaging a generationally disconnected workforce.* Published in the USA.

Marston, C. (2012). *How to train millennials.* Mobile, AL: Generational Insights.

McGillis Hall, L., LaLonde, M., Dales, L., Peterson, J., & Cripps, L. (2011). Strategies for retaining midcareer nurses. *Journal of Nursing Administration, 41*(12), 531–538.

Pettit, L. (2010). A tale of two generations. *Satisfaction Snapshot.* Press Ganey Associates. Retrieved from http:\\www.pressganey.com.au\snapshots\Tale%20of%20Two%20Generations.pdf

Pew Research Center. (2010). *Pew Social & Demographic Trends.* Pew Charitable Trust.

Quotes. Retrieved from http://thinkexist.com/quotes/with/keyword/generation/

Wieck, K. L., Dols, J., & Landrum, P. (2010). Retention priorities for the intergenerational nurse workforce. *Nursing Forum, 45*(1), 7–17.

Wisotzkey, S. (2011). Will they stay or will they go? Insight into nursing turnover. *Nursing Management 42*(2), 15–17.

6

How Does All This Impact the Patient?

If you want happiness for a lifetime,
help the next generation.
—Chinese Proverb

As you know by now, each of the four generations has a different way of doing things, from communication, to fashion statements and dress, to marriage and children. Therefore, a natural assumption arises: Generational differences between a nurse and his or her patient must somehow impact patient care.

Undoubtedly, the connection patients make with their physicians, nurses, and other caregivers strongly affects the healing environment and even patients' state of well-being.

This chapter covers:

- Patients and their relationships with their nurses and caregivers
- Health and wellness philosophies of each generation
- Nurse-patient *pairing* (matching) recommendations

Do Patients Really Care About Who Their Nurse Is?

After spending much time over the past 25 years talking to patients and their families, I believe that patients like to experience a connection with their nurses. This rapport, or even relationship, needs to include trust between both the nurse and the patient. Generally speaking, though, I don't believe that patients think much about who is taking care of them, as long as the patient feels safe and in competent hands. As with many things, however, some patients care more about who specifically is caring for them than many other patients do. Personal biases, prejudices, preconceived notions, or even cultural or religious reasons might raise patient concern about their caregivers. As a nurse manager, you want your staff to understand why patients may have these beliefs/concerns and ensure that your staff always remains caring and professional, both inside and out.

Making an Impression

This might surprise you: Even before you have fully entered a patient's room, that patient has already formed a first impression of you. This occurs regardless of patient intent and holds true for every person-to-person interaction. According to research, it takes us one-tenth of a second to make a first impression on anyone we encounter, whether a stranger or a patient (Wargo, 2006). The evidence shows that we instinctively base these judgments on facial appearance, such as eyes partially closed or open, smiling or frowning, and so on. This one-tenth-of-a-second capability has evolved over thousands of years and has served us well as a survival instinct. It turns out that this instantaneous first impression also plays a large role in how we treat others and how we get treated. I believe that this innate function plays more of an important role in what our patients think of their nurses than the generation the nurse belongs to.

> **NOTE**
>
> *As a leader, you should dress as a role model. This means clean, pressed. Professional and identifiable. This means that your identification badge is in a visible location and without pins or stickers obscuring your picture name and title. Expect the same from your staff.*

As nurses, our appearance and demeanor factor importantly here. We need to groom ourselves and dress in ways that say, "I am a professional," and "I am worthy of your trust and respect." Obviously, we want to have a welcoming look on our face, not a scowl or grimace. Be aware, as well, that appearances that patients might not expect of a nurse, such as spiked hair or multiple tattoos or piercings, may negatively influence patients' impressions. However, patients' reactions do not usually result from a lack of acceptance or tolerance, but instead from unmet expectations of what health care professionals should look like. Although this might seem somewhat stereotypical, nurses who have tattoos project less professionalism, competency, and credibility than those who do not have tattoos (as discussed earlier in this book). This fact holds true regardless of the nurse's generation.

These opinions likely derive from various formative life experiences that may cause some generations to have preconceived notions of what a nurse of a specific age or with a particular look represents to them. For example, traditionalist patients often expect nurses to wear white uniforms and doctors to wear white lab coats. Remember, however, that although some patients worry about the age or the generation of the nurse attending them, most don't care; they just want a competent nurse.

Generational Differences or Similarities?

We have discussed throughout this book the differences that each generation displays and uses to interpret behaviors, but we also need to note that similarities exist as well. The parallels are apparent through common values that run through all the generations, albeit demonstrated differently. For example, a study of physical therapy students from all four generations (traditionalists, boomers, Xers, and millennials) found that each generation considers *arriving at work on time* and *professional dress* important markers of professionalism (Gleeson, 2007). However, the different generations define these terms (professional dress and arriving at work on time) quite differently.

Consider the term *professional dress*, for example. It means different things to each of the four generations, from khaki pants and button-down shirts, to polo shirts, to shorts or track pants and T-shirts with logos. The term *arriving at work on time* means everything from arriving 15 minutes early and being ready to work to showing up "on the dot" and not technically being late.

Help young nurses understand the benefit of arriving a few minutes early, such as getting their assignment sheets in order and "mentally preparing" for their shift. In sports we call this "getting your game face on."

Another study identified similar values among 5,800 respondents born between 1925 and 1986, although the study expressed these values somewhat differently (Gleeson, 2007). In this study, all four generations highlighted the values of communication and feedback. We know that communication differs today from what it was 50 years ago. For example, words change meaning over time, and communication in recent times has become much more casual than in years past. In addition, the four generations have widely different expectations in terms of both the quantity and quality of communication. For example, traditionalists and boomers prefer a more lengthy and robust dialogue where everyone can share opinions and be heard. In contrast, Xers and millennials like short, succinct discussions that get to the point. This type of communication can seem more abbreviated or choppy and thus more casual. The popularity of communicating via texting presents yet another complexity in communication. Even though all four generations value communication and feedback, these terms have completely different meanings and are exhibited differently across all four generations.

Remember to communicate and provide feedback in a way that gets the point across clearly and in a timely manner.

Is There a Good Nurse-Patient Match?

As a result of reading this book, you now know that differences in values, characteristics, and customs may lead to misunderstanding or even generational conflict between nurses and their patients. Sometimes, unfortunately, patients may perceive these misunderstandings and misinterpretations as a lack of competence or professionalism.

When these similar but differently interpreted values are translated into the patient care environment, you can see how misunderstandings and misperceptions can occur. In a patient care situation, where a traditionalist patient has an expectation of frequent and long verbal conversations and the Xer or millennial nurse is used to providing short, abbreviated dialogue, both sides will become frustrated with the interaction. One side will not feel listened to, and the other side will not feel heard.

Another opportunity for misperceptions is the patient routine or schedule. To traditionalists and boomers, schedules are important and are meant to be adhered to; for these groups, schedules are time commitments. To Xers and millennials, however, schedules are merely placeholders and estimations. Providing traditionalist and boomer patients scheduled times for procedures or medications is important to them; they want to know what to expect and when to expect it. But, Xer and millennial nurses who must meet these time obligations find schedules constraining and rigid. When procedures and medications don't occur as scheduled, our older patients become upset and wonder about the competence of their nurse or perceive a problem. Xer and millennial nurses may have more of a laissez-faire attitude. This is but one example where the value of time, although important, has different expressions and may engender conflict between the generations.

The construct that may present the most significant challenges in patient care assignments is the acceptance of diversity. Millennials are our most traveled and diverse generation to date. This generation has been exposed to more ethnic, religious, sexual orientation, gender, educational, socioeconomic, and cultural diversity than the rest of us. You can see the perceptions forming as the broad acceptance and open-mindedness that this generation has is overlaid upon the biases and opinions that the older generations have been raised with. This is not to say that traditionalists or boomers are discriminatory or mean-spirited, but it might be hard for them to build relationships or be accepting of caregivers who differ so significantly from themselves. This is where nurse managers and nurses need to step up and introduce themselves and tell the patient a little about themselves to break down barriers and build trust.

> **NOTE**
>
> *It is important to remind staff that as nurses, we are in the customer service industry. We need to exceed our patients' (and their families') expectations with our communication skills as well as our clinical skills.*

Traditionalists, boomers, and to a much lesser degree Xers and millennials see tenure and experience as a determinant of competence and expertise. This is often true of patients more so than nurses. However, nurse managers know that this is not an accurate assumption. Our younger generations, Xers and millennials, have been educated using evidence, data, and research and can quickly access any clinical information that they are looking for and integrate it in to their practice. What they lack is the repetition of "seeing" clinical situations over and over again as our older generations of nurses have. Bridging the gap to help patients understand and appreciate the skills that these younger nurses bring to the table proves difficult sometimes. Nurse managers can help with this issue by visiting patients (or *rounding* on patients) often and speaking positively of their staff. Doing so will provide a sense of comfort to patients and their families as they hear that the nursing staff really are good clinicians and high-quality caregivers.

> **NOTE**
>
> *Teach your staff how to introduce themselves to patients so positively that the patients have confidence in their skills and expertise and feels that they are in good hands.*

Patients, too, are multigenerational and different from what they were in the past. Patients today are often highly informed consumers and much more knowledgeable than in years past. They derive much of their information from the Internet or social media. So, although the fact that patients are more knowledgeable today is generally good, sometimes the information they have does not come from reliable sources and might prove difficult to "fix." Constant patient questioning and misinformation can strain the development of the patient-caregiver relationship. Nurses (and other caregivers) may perceive the bombardment of questions as lack of trust and can feel undermined by this. This has the potential to eventually create tension for both the caregiver and the patient, which is not conducive to a strong nurse-patient relationship and may even impact patient outcomes.

> **NOTE**
>
> *It is important to educate all staff about generational differences so that they understand how to successfully navigate through them and learn not to take overly inquisitive or confrontational patients personally.*

Generational Differences and Perceptions of Wellness and Care

Today, our traditionalist patients are experiencing the aging process in earnest with sensory changes, such as vision and hearing loss, changes in taste and smell, decreased sensation to both heat and cold, and chronic illness as their bodies begin to simply wear down. Information processing and cognitive abilities are also greatly diminished among this generation, often requiring many to live in assisted-care facilities or receive regular care services (Berkowitz & Schewe, 2011). Because women outlive men by several years, many more women than men among this generation are widowed and live alone. Remember that traditionalists are the "I can survive anything" generation. They often live frugal lives because of fixed incomes and may even decline medical services or medications that are "out of pocket" because they are unable or unwilling to pay for them.

Due to how they were raised, this cohort also has a high tolerance for command and control and for authoritarian values. This implies that they generally do well with nurses who inform the patient and family of the plan and then proceed to "take charge." Generally, as caregivers, we tend to see our traditionalist, boomer, and Xer nurses do this more clearly and comfortably. As patients, the traditionalist generation is compliant and wants to follow the treatment plan, often asking few questions.

Boomers strongly believe in living a healthful lifestyle, as evidenced by their continually increasing use of health-club and gym memberships, organic foods, complementary therapies, and alternative medicines. This cohort wants to remain healthy and retain its youth as long as possible.

This desire also accounts for the increased demand in such products/treatments as Rogaine, Lasik, Viagra, and Botox.

As this generation ages, it has come to demand individuality in its senior living needs, not the cookie-cutter approach of previous assisted-living models. Boomers also are looking for different health care options than those of their parents (Berkowitz & Schewe, 2011). Boomers crave information and generally speaking are a well-informed group of health care consumers. Unlike their parents, they expect their physicians and other health care providers to partner with them in their pursuit of wellness and health.

Xers have come to expect a high personal quality of life and wellness. Throughout their lives, they have experienced adequate food supplies and grew up with fitness as a part of their regular routine. One major difference in this group's members, compared to traditionalists and boomers, is that they are typically not as accepting of long work hours and high job stress and are more than willing to make career changes to improve their own work-life balance (Berkowitz & Schewe, 2011). As discussed throughout this book, Xers are fiercely independent and as patients can fully process the information from physicians and make their own health care decisions. They are even willing to change physicians to get the treatment options that they believe best suit them.

This tech-savvy group spends hours on websites, blogs, and social media to understand diagnoses, treatments, and care options as well as physician and hospital quality metrics. It is not unheard of for Xers, when faced with an illness, to show up to a physician's office with a significant amount of research already in hand, prepared to discuss medications or treatment options. They are also willing to travel to find what they consider the highest quality of care for them or their loved ones. This group does not like to be told what to do but rather prefers treatment choices and options and participating in the decision making. This is seen in hospitalized Xers as well as those who visit physicians in their offices. Some health care providers might misinterpret this behavior as noncompliance, but it is in fact a need for more information and participation in the process.

As you know by now, millennials are our most wired generation thus far (not considering the yet-unnamed generation). This group can use its smartphones to "Google" any medication or treatment option at lightning speed (Berkowitz & Schewe, 2011). Being educated in an evidence-based world has made this group efficient at accessing data and using information. Members often make their health care choices based on feedback from online sources and from word of mouth. This cohort is satisfied with meeting with physician extenders if doing so meets with its demand for convenience, such as shorter wait times and easier access. Millennials are also willing to have e-mail "conversations" with physicians or video chats instead of in-person office visits.

You can readily see how the perceptions of health care and wellness have changed through the generations and over time.

NOTE

Overall our patients are more informed today regarding medical issues and treatments. We need to ensure that our nurses are better educated than our patients. This may mean ongoing education for your staff, via journal articles, computer-based learning, or in-services from experts to remain current.

Pairing or Matching Patients and Their Nurses

Matching patients and nurses is more of an art than a science, with no particular right way or wrong way to match them. To facilitate any matching, nurses must work hard to meet the needs of their patients, regardless of age or generation (of the caregiver or the patient). Table 6.1 provides some thought-provoking guideline generalizations.

As mentioned earlier, generally speaking there is no right way or a wrong way to assign patients to their nurse caregivers; and so, to some degree, one could argue that this chapter is an oversimplification. However, this chapter is based on the literature and evidence reviewed for this book. Patient assignments should be based on individual patient needs and specific nurse skills and capabilities. Developing positive relationships with caregivers represents an important part of the healing and wellness process. Both patients and nurses have the ability to establish a good relationship with anyone of any generation, race, religion, or background as long as they remain receptive and willing to do so.

Summary

Patients benefit when they have a *good relationship* with their nurses—that is, a strong person-to-person connection between the patient and nurse based on trust, competency, and respect. Nurse managers can facilitate this by maintaining a competent workforce, rounding on their patients, "talking up" their staff, and building relationships with patients and their families to solicit feedback.

TABLE 6.1
NURSE: PATIENT PAIRING MATRIX

	Traditionalist Nurse	Boomer Nurse	Xer Nurse	Millennial Nurse
Traditionalist Patient	Good match: They can relate to each other and understand each other's care and communication needs.	Generally a good match.	May be comfortable or awkward, depends more on personality or relationship fit.	Millennial nurses often perceive multitasking as preoccupation or not willing to take the time these patients need. These nurses may provide less human contact and seem less caring. However, millennials often affectionately view traditionalists as grandparent-like.
Boomer Patient	Good match: They respect their elders and will therefore respect their older caregivers.	Good match: They can relate to each other and understand each other's care and communication needs.	May be comfortable or awkward, depends more on personality or relationship fit.	May have a parent-like relationship with these patients because they remind them of their own parents. Comfortable relationship.
Xer Patient	Xer patients may view traditionalists as less flexible and not as resourceful (based on the need for online information).	May be comfortable or awkward, depends more on personality or relationship fit.	Good match: They can relate to each other and understand each other's care and communication needs.	Xers don't like to be outperformed by these rivals, who in their opinion are using entitlements regularly in their lives. They might also envy the Xer's willingness to live more simply for a better work-life balance.
Millennial Patient	May or may not be a good match. Millennials often affectionately view traditionalists as grandparent-like, but may become frustrated at a lack of interest in multitasking and Internet culture.	May have a parent-child relationship with these patients because they remind them of their own children. Comfortable relationship.	May or may not be a good match. Xers might envy the millennial's willingness to live more simply for a better work-life balance.	Good match: They can relate to each other and understand each other's care and communication needs.

Patients typically do not get to choose their nurses, and nurses usually do not get to choose their patients. However, we still provide care for hundreds of thousands of patients each year. To make this care effective, both sides must communicate with respect and be open-minded about each other.

As a nurse manager, you have many competing priorities each and every day, none more important than the outcomes of your patients. So, educate your staff about how to handle patients who might be less than thrilled with who is caring for them that shift. Nurses always need to take the high road and provide the best care possible to every patient, every day. Keep your staff engaged and communicate with them often. Together you can do this!

References

Berkowitz, E. N., & Schewe, C. D. (2011). Generational cohorts hold the key to understanding patients and health care providers: Coming of age experiences influence health care behaviors for a lifetime. *Health Marketing Quarterly*, 28, 190–204.

Gleeson, P. B. (2007). Understanding generational competence related to professionalism: Misunderstandings that lead to a perception of unprofessional behavior. *Journal of Physical Therapy Education*, 21(3).

Wargo, E. (2006). How many seconds to a first impression? Observer, 19(7). Retrieved from http://www.psychologicalscience.org/index.php/publications/observer/2006/july-06/how-many-seconds-to-a-first-impression.html

7

Conclusions

Raising children is an incredibly hard and risky business
in which no cumulative wisdom is gained: each generation
repeats the mistakes the previous one made.
–Bill Cosby

As you have learned throughout this book, generational
differences are apparent in anything and everything staff
related, including recruitment, retention, orientation,
communication, staff development, and succession
planning. After reviewing all the information in this book
about how we have all been influenced during our formative
years, you should now better understand these generational
differences. This understanding will help you assist each
individual on your staff to reach his or her full potential.

This chapter covers:

- Integrating the concepts of generational variation in performance management, succession planning, recruitment, and retention

- Creating a generational development plan

Generational differences should not be ignored. Instead, they should be discussed and even celebrated. In fact, the American Organization of Nurse Executives (AONE) acknowledged generational differences in its strategic plan, indicating that "recognizing the impact of generational differences, it is necessary to foster the development of aspiring, novice and future nurse leaders to position and prepare them to be leaders in the design and adoption of future delivery models" (AONE, 2011). This is an opportunity for us to learn more about how each other works and how we can build a culture of acceptance and tolerance in the workplace.

The millennials comprise the fifteenth generation of Americans thus far, with the most recent, unnamed generation becoming our sixteenth (Strauss & Howe, 1991). As you now know, each generation is different and has a different perspective, point of reference, set of values, thought processes, and way of doing things. Your knowledge of generational differences will help you, as a nursing manager, to reduce misunderstandings, minimize generational conflict, and maximize the likelihood that your department will successfully achieve its goals.

To help you navigate through our current complex workforce, I have summed up five very general key action points for you. These should act as a guide for you when managing an intergenerational workforce. Review these and use them to help plan and guide your staff interactions.

TIP

If something happened before 2001, it's not worth the time to recap for millennials. That is a lifetime ago and makes you appear old. Older people like history; it makes us interesting and valuable. Young people don't see it that way; it appears dated (Satran, 2009).

Key Action Point 1: Know the Generations

Nurse managers need to learn as much as possible about the four generations in the current workplace. You might not always agree with the differences, and you might want each generation to act within your frame of reference and comfort, but you may need to compromise. In addition to increasing your own understanding, you need to spend the time educating your staff about generational differences. Gradually increase the knowledge base of everyone in your department; otherwise, tension, misunderstanding, and conflict may arise from the various generations' not "getting" each other. An intergenerational workforce requires mutual participation on everyone's part to ensure a culture of respect, tolerance, and acceptance. Put simply, shed light on the differences but avoid the stereotypes.

NOTE

Seventy-six percent of baby boomers participate in defined contribution plans, 33% of Gen Xers participate, and 50% of millennials contribute (Aon Hewitt, 2010).

Key Action Point 2: Speak the "Language" of Your Staff

Nurse managers need to take the time to learn the best way to communicate with each generation. This means that you will have to modify or "translate" the message for each of the generational cohorts. You will have to experiment with staff meetings, e-mails, group texts, and websites until you find which combination of these optimizes your staff communication. This includes knowing the mode and frequency of communication that is the most effective with each group. The goal here should be over communication.

> The average rate of savings is 5.3% of pay for millennials, 6.8% of pay for Gen Xers, and 8% of pay for baby boomers (Aon Hewitt, 2010).

Another important part of effectively communicating is listening. Allowing your staff to share their perspective and creativity in problem solving opens the door to improved staff engagement and satisfaction, which sets the stage for high-quality patient care. It takes time to change how you are used to communicating, but this is an important skill to master.

Key Action Point 3: Customize Performance Management and Succession Planning

Nurse managers want to become skilled at developing innovative and creative ways to individualize coaching for staff performance improvement. You should strive to increase employee motivation and engagement so that your entire unit/department is working toward the same organizational goals and enjoying the journey. In addition, you want to make sure that you have a well-thought-out succession plan for your key positions so that the

> *Six out of ten millennials cash out their 401(k) when they change employers, almost half of Gen Xers cash out (Aon Hewitt, 2010).*

success of your department can continue in the long term. However, just as important as the plan is the process of how you will identify and match mentors. Finally, the ongoing coaching and development of your future leaders will ensure that they have the skills necessary to step into vacant key positions as soon as you need them.

Key Action Point 4: Know Who You Are Recruiting and Retaining

The current workforce consists of traditionalists, who are eligible to retire; boomers, who are nearing retirement (many of whom are eligible now; Xers, who want to work less and live more; and millennials, who want less responsibility and a meaningful life. The challenge facing health care, just like in all industries, is how to keep our potential retirees as long as possible while continuing to attract young, new talent.

As a nurse manager recruiting for vacant positions, you need to know who you are recruiting. If you are looking for Xers, you need to be prepared to aggressively offer what is important to them: flexible schedules, vacation time, professional-growth opportunities, advancement opportunities, and so on. For each generation, you have to use the right tactics to attract its members to your department.

Keeping your employees is as important, or even more important, than finding new ones. As you have learned throughout this book, certain strategies "speak" to each generation's needs and desires, so you want to pursue retention from this perspective. Be creative and try to provide what each group cannot live without: Is it recognition, time off to volunteer, or changing schedules each year for school-age children? You will have to figure it out and determine how to appropriately meet these needs to keep your team together.

Key Action Point 5: Implement Your Plan

The nurse manager's influence establishes and maintains the overall climate and culture of the department. What you permit, you promote. You have the ability to create a positive environment just as easily as a negative one. A workplace where all the generations can maximize their strengths and contribute their creative and innovative ideas will benefit the department/unit.

Embrace the diversity of your department and create a culture that encourages individuality (within acceptable ranges) and generational harmony. You will find that this improves teamwork, engagement, and retention and ultimately improves patient care and safety. Allowing your staff to make their contributions in their own way shows them that you value what they bring to the department. After all, we need to move past the traditional "this is how we do it here" mentality and become more receptive to new ways of doing things. Encourage participation in departmental evidence-based practice or quality-improvement groups to allow for shared decision making, which is a necessary pillar of a high-retention environment.

The fortune that I found recently in a fortune cookie humorously depicts what many of us know already (Figure 7.1): Changes occur throughout all our lives. So, it is important to remember that we are not all working from the same values baseline.

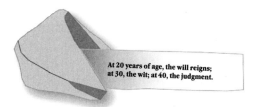

At 20 years of age, the will reigns; at 30, the wit; at 40, the judgment.

FIGURE 7.1

Keep Your Plan Simple

An easy way to manage the planning and implementation process is to utilize an annual generational development plan. I find that this simple tool helps keep me on track. The key concepts discussed in every chapter of this book are highlighted on the left side of this table (Topic Area); it also helps capture the audience, the actions that I am going to take, who is responsible, and my time line. This is an example so you can see how my planing tool would look. This breaks your plans into "bite-sized" actions, so that it is not so daunting and you can see your progress. It is important to remember that you cannot do this alone; it requires your entire leadership team as well as your staff to work together to change the culture of your department. Delegate appropriately and enlist the help of your supervisors/charge nurses, as much of this can be handled by them. This plan can be revised collectively with your leadership team once each year.

Topic Area	Audience	Actions	Responsible	Time Line
Generational Education	All unit-based staff	Education via in-services and staff meetings	Nurse manager	One topic each month
Communication Differences	All staff	E-mail out staff meeting minutes or notices, text staff meeting reminders to staff. Post short "important information" in bathrooms and by time clock each week.	Nurse manager Supervisors Charge nurses	Ongoing
Transition/Orientation	Preceptors	Annual preceptor training, including a focus on generation learning styles	Educators to train preceptors	All current unit-based preceptors to go through refresher this calendar year
Performance Management	All staff	Provide individualized coaching opportunities at annual evaluation and as appropriate opportunities arise.	Nurse manager Supervisors Charge nurses	Should be ongoing to optimize staff performance
Succession Plan	High performers Staff who have expressed interest in leadership	Leadership team to identify high performers interested in assuming leadership responsibilities in future	Nurse manager Supervisors Charge nurses	Identify potential candidates at least annually at evaluation time

Recruitment Plan	Applicant pool	Implement self-scheduling model. Work with recruiters to identify applicant pool, target group with specific generational scheduling needs.	Nurse manager	Six months for self-governance council to help develop scheduling revisions Implement in recruitment collaterals as soon as ready
Retention Plan	Existing staff	Identify some targeted retention tactics for group with highest risk to leave. Implement a change at a time.	Nurse manager Supervisors Charge nurses	Work through self-governance council to help develop innovative (or even previously recycled) ideas
Patient-Satisfaction Opportunities	Patients All staff	Round on patients and share feedback with staff. Use any trends in patient assignments to help craft future assignments.	Nurse manager Supervisors Charge nurses All staff	Ongoing

FIGURE 7.2

Annual Generational Development Plan

Final Remarks

I hope that this book has given you some new things to think about and some tools to help you become a more effective intergenerational leader. It is important for leaders at all levels of the organization to understand the differences that each generation brings to the workplace so that all the diversity, creativity, and energy can be channeled into making the organization successful in its overall mission, vision, and goals. Now that you better understand generational differences, you will find it both challenging and rewarding to implement some of these newly learned tactics. Remember that you cannot change how your staff are "wired" but you can become more effective in managing them.

Understanding generational differences while providing for workforce demands is a difficult balancing act. Nurse managers should learn to leverage generational strengths and create a workplace of respect, acceptance, and generational harmony. While pursuing the goals of the department, and to promote a workplace where a culture of retention thrives, the nurse manager should make it an overall goal to provide each employee with what he or she needs. The current workforce is looking for its own version of career development, meaningful work, professional growth, and development and work-life balance. As long as you remain flexible and adaptable, you and your staff will succeed. Don't be shy, be creative.

Best of luck, and enjoy yourself. Managing the intergenerational workforce can be fun!

–Bonnie

References

AONE. American Organization of Nurse Executives. (2011, December). AONE supports the Institute of Medicine's recommendations on the future of nursing. Retrieved from http://nurseleader.com

Aon Hewitt. (2010). Retirement readiness: Bridging the gap across generations study. Chicago, IL. Hewitt & Associates.

Satran, P. (2009). *How not to act old*. New York: HarperCollins Publishers.

Strauss, W., & Howe, N. (1991). *Generations: The history of America's future, 1584–2069*. New York: Quill Publishing.

Index